The Quintessence Tantras of Tibetan Medicine

To Laney,

wishing you the
bliss of the
Medicine Buddha,

[signature]

The Quintessence Tantras of Tibetan Medicine

Foreword by H.H. the Dalai Lama
Translated by Dr. Barry Clark

Snow Lion Publications
Ithaca, New York USA

Snow Lion Publications
P.O. Box 6483
Ithaca, New York 14851
USA

Printed in USA.

ISBN 1-55939-009-3

Library of Congress Cataloging-in-Publication Data

Rgyud bźi. Rtsa rgyud. English
    Quintessence tantras of Tibetan medicine / foreword by
H.H. the Dalai Lama ; translated by Barry Clark.
        p. cm.
    Includes index.
    ISBN 1-55939-009-3
    1. Rgyud bźi. 2. Medicine, Tibetan. I. Clark, Barry, 1949-
II. Rgyud bźi. Man nag rgyud stod cha. English. 1992.
R127.5.R49513 1995
615.5'3--dc20   93-40282
                                                                CIP

Contents

THE DALAI LAMA

FOREWORD

I am happy that after more than ten years studying Tibetan medicine, both in theory and practice under the tutelage of a number of reputable Tibetan physicians, Barry Clark has compiled this book, **The Quintessence Tantra**. In it he presents clear and accurate translations of the Root and Explanatory Tantras, two works of such fundamental importance in the Tibetan medical system that they are commonly memorised by medical students.

Tibetan medicine is an integrated system of health care that has served the Tibetan people well for many centuries and which, I believe, can still provide much benefit to humanity at large. The difficulty we face in bringing this about is one of communication, for, like other scientific systems, Tibetan medicine must be understood in its own terms, as well as in the context of objective investigation. Barry Clark is making a great contribution in this direction. He has been careful to express Tibetan medical terms in language that is accurate in its identification of scientific terminology and accessible to the English reader. I am sure his work will be of immense benefit for serious students of Tibetan medicine, as well as providing an opportunity for general readers to appreciate another valuable aspect of the Tibetan cultural heritage.

Dedication
To my daughters, Nicola and Monique,
for their outstanding courage.

Translator's Introduction

Our world is crying out for remedies to universal malaises and maladies, not the least of which take the form of serious diseases which are often impossible to cure.

The remedies and treatments found in the ancient Tibetan medical system have been overlooked for many centuries, but it is important that they should not continue to be disregarded. This is because these treatments are now more widely available than before, and because the advent of new incurable syndromes necessitates seeking cures from valid sources, including the most ancient ones. In an endeavor at least to open doors to revolutionary, natural cures for the mental and physical ills of mankind, I have translated two medical tantras and produced this book.

According to Tibetan history, the first mention of Tibetan medicine is found in an eighth-century text by the Indian Adept Acharya Padmasambhava. This work describes how the Tibetans discovered the divine being Nya.tri Tsan.po, and since they considered him to have descended to earth from a celestial realm, they invited him to be their king. At the time, to remove his qualms, they assured him that they possessed the means to overcome various obstacles and afflictions, including medicines to overcome diseases.

Other sources suggest that what we now know as the Tibetan medical system has existed in the universe for the inconceivably long timespan of fifty aeons. This would mean that for as long as there has been humanoid life in the universe with the three humors or three-fold division of bodily energy, so there has existed a medical tradition to heal imbalances or disorders of the three humors.

The commonly accepted historical account of 'Tibetan Medicine' is that it was the ancient system of medicine taught by an emanation of the historical Buddha, and practiced extensively throughout the length and breadth of the vast empire of King Asoka in a network of welfare dispensaries, before being transmitted and propagated in Tibet along with Lord Buddha's spiritual teachings.

As the Buddhist doctrine went into decline in the Indian subcontinent and was transmitted to Tibet, the four medical tantras were also propagated and translated there by the Indian pandit Chandrananda and the Tibetan translator Vairochana in the eighth century C.E. To ensure their survival, the tantras were concealed as a 'treasure text' in a pillar in Samye Monastery until the time was ripe for them to be revealed and fully propagated.

Although there are indications of a simpler medical tradition based on the 'Eight Branches' dating from ancient times in Tibet, it was only with the advent of the Buddha's teachings that the country acquired a more evolved, profound and elaborate medical system. Now, more than a thousand years later, one of the greatest gifts that Tibetan culture has to offer the world is its advanced medical system preserved through the ages with remarkable and pristine purity. In fact this medical system has been 'tried and tested' for thousands of years and its proven ability to stand the test of time testifies to its efficacy. Some may say that having as its origin an infallible, enlightened source is adequate testimony of the value of Tibetan medicine. However, in addition to this, in the last three decades, as Tibetan medicine has taken root 'in exile,' many thousands of people all over the world have experienced remarkable relief and cures of a vast range of both physical and mental disorders. Another attractive feature of the system is its wide range of non-chemical drugs, compounded from natural substances of plant and mineral origin, and possessing a therapeutic action completely free from side effects in almost all cases.

The entire syllabus for Tibetan medical study comprises four traditionally esoteric works or 'tantras,' in which all aspects of the system are expounded in detail. The present work comprises the first two of these works, the Root Tantra and the Explanatory Tantra. Especially impressive and revealing is the third work, the Oral Instruction Tantra, which provides extensive explanation of the causes, conditions, classifications, diagnosis, symptoms and treatments of a very wide range of disease syndromes, in a lengthy span of ninety-two chapters. The fourth and so-called 'Final Tantra' completes the detailed presentation of the entire medical system and contains two extensive chapters on the principles of pulse and urine diagnosis, followed by a lengthy series of chapters presenting various different types of medicinal compounds as well as numerous pacification, evacuation and accessory therapies. The vastness and complexity of the Oral Instruction and Final Tantras accounts for the absence of an English translation of these until now.

Traditionally the long and rigorous training of a Tibetan physician commenced when he had barely entered his teens, and included the memorization of all one hundred and fifty-six chapters of the four tantras as well as training in being able to identify dozens, even hundreds, of different medicinal plants simply by tasting them while blindfolded. After at least six or seven years of theoretical training followed by two years under the guidance of an experienced practitioner, one became a full-fledged graduate physician. For many aspirants the path to becoming a Tibetan physician has proved arduous and fraught with obstacles. I too recall experiencing prolonged periods of malnutrition in the early years of my study, and still I have far to go until I achieve my teachers' inspiring diagnostic abilities which to many patients appear to be nothing short of clairvoyance.

Even a casual investigation of the principles and practice of Tibetan medicine will reveal a medical system which is unique in many respects and strikingly different from other systems including Ayurveda, with which it has nonetheless a number of noteworthy parallels. For example, both Tibetan medicine and Ayurveda have in common the *tridosa* system of the three 'humors' or divisions of bodily energy. However, the extremely

detailed presentation of foetus development and urine diagnosis are unique to Tibetan medicine alone. One important
premise of Tibetan medicine is that even the so-called healthy
human organism is not intrinsically healthy at all.

Since the three humors - wind, bile and phlegm - are rooted
in attachment, hatred and obscuration respectively, they are
considered to be contaminated, impure factors, acting as a
target or 'magnetic' basis which attracts and receives afflictions.
Thus the disturbed or imbalanced humors become the very
nature of disease rather than its cause. The objects of harm or
targets which are struck are the branch-humors, physical
constituents and excretions. The actual cause of the arisal of
disease may be any of the following four: season, spirit, dietary
and behavioral factors; whilst the disease uses as its means of
entry the skin, flesh, channels, bones, vital and vessel organs
in turn. Finally the individual organs and bodily constituents act
both as pathways of arisal and specific locations of the disorder.
In addition to these, certain natural rising periods of disease
according to seasonal changes, etc. are presented as well as a
number of fatal syndromes and reaction imbalances. The most
fundamental division of disorders is into hot and cold, thus
distinguishing between blood and bile disorders on the one
hand, and wind and phlegm on the other. The only conditions
which may be either hot or cold in nature are parasitic and
lymphatic disorders.

The ancient and profound diagnostic techniques of Tibetan
medicine have long been a source of wonderment to patients
the world over. Years ago during a private audience His
Holiness the Dalai Lama commented to me that a skilled
Tibetan doctor can through pulse diagnosis ascertain features
of a patient's condition which whole laboratories of modern
equipment could never find.

Indeed the ability of experienced Tibetan physicians to
discover a patient's symptoms and medical history purely
through palpation is strongly reminiscent of extra-sensory
perception. Apart from visual diagnosis using the tongue, the
first two chapters of the final tantra present in detail the
principles of pulse and urine diagnosis. The use of these,
together with the actual questioning of the patient, enable the
physician to build up a composite picture of the patient's

condition. On this basis treatment is prescribed traditionally in a graded manner, integrating dietary and behavioral factors with formal medication.

Around 300 C.E. one early Greek traveller to India noted that the physicians of that time treated disease using a wide range of different foods in much the same way as doctors use medicines nowadays. In extreme cases where various types of medicinal compounds in the form of pills, powders, decoctions, concentrates, extracts, oils, etc. prove inadequate to cure a disorder, appropriate powerful accessory therapies, such as venesection, moxabustion, fomentation, massage, etc. are applied.

With respect to the knowledge and use of raw drugs of plant and mineral origin, Tibetan medicine really comes into its own. Nowadays only very few animal products are used, although many are documented in the traditional texts. Apart from a total pharmacopoeia of well over two thousand compounds, the system contains a materia medica of several thousand gem, mineral and plant medicines. Prior to the Chinese Communist invasion of Tibet in the 1950s, thousands of medical texts were extant in Tibet, but in the last forty years the majority of these have been lost. There remain a few texts both ancient and modern which expound in detail the properties and uses of Tibetan materia medica. Undoubtedly the greatest surviving text in this category is the *Crystal Orb* with its auto-commentary, *Crystal Rosary*, composed circa 1737 by the great Tibetan scholar Dilmar Geshe Tenzin Phuntsok. This and similar texts document thousands of gem, plant, mineral and animal medicines according to which of the six tastes, eight natural potencies, three post-digestive 'tastes,' seventeen secondary qualities and individual uses each possesses.

The actual compounding of Tibetan medicines is probably the most advanced and secret aspect of the whole system: the Tibetan physician has by tradition and necessity always been his or her own pharmacologist, and in order to compound one single drug he or she has to be cognizant with the tastes, natural potencies, post-digestive factors, secondary qualities and uses of each of several dozen different ingredients. Moreover he or she has to be skilled in the preparation of the relevant part of each plant, etc. and experienced in the compounding of medicines using the correct ratios of the individual ingredients according to the traditional prescribed Tibetan weights and measures. Without thorough training in all the above aspects, it is practically impossible for an outsider to compound an authentic Tibetan medicine.

I have often found it strange to hear outsiders dismiss the medicinal properties ascribed to plants and herbs in their natural form as superstition or 'hocus-pocus.' Since a great number of allopathic drugs contain products synthesized from plants, etc. it is absurdly illogical to deny that the latter have any medicinal uses in their raw state. Such intellectual arrogance hardly compensates for a lack of awareness of ancient knowledge.

One account in particular from the time of the Buddha himself illustrates the far-reaching holistic view of this ancient Buddhist medical system. According to different versions, the master-physician in the story is either the Buddha himself or his personal physician, Jivaka.

One day the Master asked his disciples to go out into the country and bring back with them anything and everything they could find which was not medicine. Within a few hours most of them had returned, bearing a few apparently useless plant or mineral substances. By the end of the day all the disciples except one had returned carrying something of apparently no medicinal value. It was only after several days that the last disciple appeared, weary, dust stained and ... empty handed. He explained humbly to the Master, "I looked far and wide, but I could find nothing at all which is not a medicine." The Master congratulated and praised him warmly for having been the only trainee to realize the medicinal value of all material things.

Nowadays we have a far greater range of natural and synthetic substances available in the world. Only the true wisdom to realize their medicinal potential is lacking.

Undoubtedly the most powerful medicinal substances used in Tibetan medicine are precious gems and metals. The most complete exposition of these is found in the *Crystal Rosary*. Precious gems such as diamond, aquamarine, sapphire, ruby and emerald are said to protect against spirits, and to cure all diseases (when compounded in medicine). Their various sub-types are described very clearly in the above text and their values quoted in terms of the combined resources of the number of provinces, countries and even world systems that each is worth. Allowing for the increased rarity of the most precious types and the rate of inflation over the last two hundred and fifty years since these original estimates were given, their value nowadays must be inestimable. For those who have long wondered and sought, *Crystal Rosary* identifies and describes even the precious 'wish-fulfilling gem' as being generally yellow in color and bearing a design of seven eyes formed of five different colors. Two means of testing the authenticity of this gem are explained: if one wraps it in several layers of cloth, and offers a prayer of truth over it, the gem will appear on the surface of the cloth without puncturing it. Secondly if one looks through the gem at the sky, even in bright sunlight, one can see the light of every star. Its original value is stated to be that of the combined wealth of the world.

Even a number of eminent plant substances are said to have sacred or celestial origins. The accounts of chebulic myrobalan, saffron, sandalwood, etc. suggest that some of them were transplanted from celestial realms or distant lands to certain countries by gods, dakinis, sages and spiritually realized beings for the future benefit of humanity.

By the time this book goes to press, I hope to have been able correctly to identify most, if not all, of the substances described in the materia medica and other chapters of the Explanatory Tantra. In the past thirteen years I have consulted a wide range of medical and botanical works in the Tibetan, Sanskrit, English, Hindi, Chinese, French, Russian and Mongolian languages. The data given in some of these is occasionally suspect and it has not been possible to undertake sufficiently extensive field trips to collect and identify all the substances listed. Nonetheless over many years I have consulted many eminent scholars, physicians, botanists, geologists and zoologists in India, Tibet, Nepal, Hong Kong and England. For the purpose of this research I have visited museums, universities, herbariums and botanical gardens, and accompanied teams of Tibetan doctors, students and botanists on plant collecting expeditions, sometimes climbing up to sixteen thousand feet in the mountains of the Himalayas and Tibet. I regret that occasionally when the rain was too heavy or the snows too deep, I was forced to leave a few stones (and alpine herbs) unturned. Also a small number of pressed plant specimens and photographic prints and slides remain to be identified.

Whilst many precious medicinal plants have become so rare as to be almost extinct, and the identity of others is shrouded in obscurity, still many herbs and raw drugs having remarkable properties are available. Some of these such as Round-leaf Sundew, and the roots of Angelica, Polygonatum and Salep orchid have exceptional fortifying and rejuvenating properties. The latter root was even popular in eighteenth-century London as a tonic infusion. These as well as certain flowers and types of calcite and mineral exudate have long been renowned also in the preparation of 'essence-extraction' compounds, which apart from their invigorating qualities enable meditators and yogis to live without intake of gross food and thus engage in spiritual practices with enhanced mental clarity, sharpness and pliancy.

Whilst the Tibetan medical system in the most literal sense is allopathic in healing by means of 'other,' i.e. force opposite in nature to the disease, it also contains elements of the 'doctrine of signatures' as propounded by Paracelsus. This principle has long been exemplified throughout the world in the phenomena of fruits, roots, seeds, etc. having the shape of a specific organ of the body and having a therapeutic action on that same organ. Other medicinal substances function according to the same principle by having a different factor (e.g., color) in common with the type of the disorder which they treat. Prominent examples of the above principles are the three *zho.sha* fruits which are shaped like and named after the kidney, spleen and heart. These three are identified respectively as *Canavalia gladiata, Entada scandens* and *Spondias axillans*, and just as they are used to treat disorders of the correspondingly shaped organs, so for example, the yellow cambium of Indian Barberry is used to treat bilious disorders. In this latter case the bitter taste of the plant also makes it efficacious in the treatment of such disorders. Similarly the tastes, powers, etc. of the other substances covered by this principle often support or even surpass the 'doctrine of signatures' in their therapeutic action.

Whilst the compounding of Tibetan medicines is carried out

with great precision, so also precise guidelines are laid down for their collection in the *Crystal Rosary*, Final Tantra and other tantric texts. Herbs should be collected from fertile areas and not from areas shaded by very large trees nor from built-up areas or the environs of a cemetery. Cool-powered plants should be collected from north-facing slopes where they receive much shade, and warm-powered ones should be collected from south-facing valleys. Such plants should have large deep roots and should be undamaged by insects or the elements. Generally roots should be collected in the spring; flowers, leaves, stalks, seedlings and whole herbs in the monsoon season; and bark, resin and roots in the spring. The recommended time for collection is on auspicious days during the waxing phase of the moon, especially from the seventh to fifteenth days of the lunar month when all such substances 'turn to nectar.' Traditionally herb collection should be formally commenced by a freshly bathed child of six or seven years wearing ornaments and white clothing. Moreover collection should be accompanied by recitation of the mantra of the Medicine Buddha or the mantra of the 'Essence of Dependent Arising.'

Within a few days of being collected the plants should be beaten, e.g., with sticks, in order to retain their power, smell and taste, for if they are simply dried without this treatment they will become like pale, dry straw devoid of their original tastes and potencies. Cool-powered plants should be dried in the shade, and warm-powered ones in the sun or near a fire. Finally, collected plants may be stored for up to one year but should not be compounded if they are older than that. Once compounded into pills the latter may be stored for two years or more, especially if their surface is sealed and coated.

Considered in its entirety the state of Tibetan Medicine in the world today cannot be said to be flourishing and the practice of this system is limited largely to Tibet, Nepal, India and Mongolia, and in particular to the Himalayan regions. Along with the rest of Tibetan culture, Tibetan medicine suffered almost total destruction at the hands of the Chinese for many years before being revived. Its centers of learning and for the training of new doctors are very few, and between them they produce a maximum of only a few dozen graduate doctors every few years. Most of the great and gifted physicians of this tradition are advanced in years and the preservation of the textual tradition has largely been left to one public-spirited physician from Ladakh and to those whose lives and work are under the rigid control of the Chinese in Tibet. Not surprisingly, only a mere fraction of the previously vast corpus of Tibetan medical treatises remains extant.

The nature of tantra is traditionally esoteric and hidden, and in this regard the medical tantras are no different from those tantras which contain advanced and secret meditation techniques. In preparing this translation, therefore, I have interpolated liberally from the *Blue Aquamarine* commentary in order correctly to interpret and accurately render many passages. In order to bring out the full meaning of the root texts I have also relied on oral teachings.

Phonetic renderings of Sanskrit names were obtained from Tibetan texts and other sources, and since many of these names are not to be found even in the largest available Sanskrit dictionaries, diacritics have been omitted from Sanskrit terms and names for the sake of consistency. For this reason too the Sanskrit equivalents of many Tibetan names could not be traced and therefore are only included where available.

All outlines are presented exactly as in the root texts, except that headings have been added, and, for example, in chapter two of the Root Tantra very brief summaries of a number of chapters have been interpolated in parentheses to afford the reader a glimpse of the unique Tibetan approach to various syndromes and treatments. These interpolations are based on Dr. Yeshe Donden's teachings on the Oral Instruction and other tantras. Interpolations in square brackets [ ] are taken from the *Blue Aquamarine* commentary and *Spreading Tree* commentary, whilst those in parentheses ( ) are derived from the oral instructions of Dr. Yeshe Donden and Dr. Pema Dorje. Examples of types of medicines used in chapter five of the Root Tantra were taken from the *Spreading Tree* commentary.

In the twentieth chapter of the Explanatory Tantra on materia medica I have presented first the Tibetan name of each substance as a precise reference for scholars. This is because a great deal of Tibetan materia medica has remained either totally unidentified or only tentatively identified, and so many scholars will be familiar only with the Tibetan names of these substances. Thereafter I have given each entry an English name where available and in almost all cases it is followed by at least one scientific name. Often more than one identification is available and sometimes the same name refers to different plants growing in unrelated geographical locations. Therefore more than one Latin name is frequently given for one substance. Where any doubt at all remains regarding the identity of certain animal products the Tibetan names have been included in parentheses with the probable English identification.

ACKNOWLEDGMENTS

My deepest heartfelt thanks are due to the late Dr. Kunga Phuntsok for his inspiration, limitless kindness and help especially during the months I spent with him in Lhasa, Tibet in 1987. Throughout his eighty-six years he supremely embodied all the teachings of the Medicine Buddha. My deepest heartfelt gratitude is also due to Dr. Yeshe Donden, my teacher of eighteen years, who trained me with the kindness of the Medicine Buddha himself and who answered countless questions to enable me to clarify many points in the medicine tantras. To Dr. Pema Dorje, my first teacher, who instructed me almost daily for seven years, I express my profound gratitude, for his unfailing kindness, and patience in answering my manifold questions on the meaning of the tantras. Warmest thanks are also due to my friends and mentors Dr. Toding Rinpoche, Dr. Pasang Yonten, and also Dr. Tsewang Tamdin for spending many hours with me dissecting the meanings of the tantras and their commentaries. I am also extremely indebted to Professor Jyotir Mitra, head of the department of Basic Principles of the faculty of Ayurveda at Benares Hindu University, Uttar Pradesh, for his diligent and enthusiastic appraisal of the present work, and to Dr. V.K. Joshi of the Dravyaguna department of the same university for his help in identifying Sanskrit materia medica. My thanks also to Mr. Pen Ghao Jao, Botany Lecturer at the University of Lhasa, and Mr. Yung Sai Cheong of the Chinese University of Hong Kong for help in identifying plants in the materia medica section of the Explanatory Tantra.

As one eminent Tibetan physician recently suggested to an

assembly of foreign students, "The task of unearthing and revealing the treasures of Tibetan medicine cannot be accomplished by one man alone. It requires the combined 'spadework' of many people" (to assist in this). It is my fervent prayer that all interest generated by the publication of the present work may lead to this 'treasure' being shared throughout the world.

24th December 1988
Dr. Barry Clark
Dhargye Buddhist Centre
22 Royal Terrace
Dunedin
New Zealand

PART ONE

THE ROOT TANTRA

The Quintessence Tantra: The Secret Oral Tradition of the
Eight Branches of the Science of Healing

Sanskrit: *Amrta hrdayaanga astaguhyaupadesa tantra*

Tibetan:
bDud.rtsi.snying.po.yan.lag.brgyad.pa.gsang.ba.man.ngag.gi.rgyud

Obeisance by Pandit and Translator

1. Introduction

I prostrate to the king of Aquamarine Light, Master of Medicine, the perfectly accomplished Awakened One, Foe Destroyer and fully endowed transcendent Conqueror who has thus gone (beyond). By virtue of his compassion those who hear merely the name of this transcendent, accomplished Subduer, who acts to benefit living beings, are protected from the miseries of evil states of existence. I prostrate to the Aquamarine Light, the Master of Medicine and Awakened One who dispels the three poisons and [three] ailments. Thus I have spoken at one time (because both masters are emanations of the Lord of Medicine).

In the City of Medicine, an abode of sages called 'Beautiful to Behold,' lies a palace made from the five types of precious substances. This palace is adorned with various kinds of precious gems for healing the four hundred and four diseases which arise from disorders of wind, bile, phlegm and from combinations of two or all three humors. Moreover, they cool fever, warm cold disorders, pacify the one thousand and eighty types of obstacles [to good health] and fulfil all needs and desires.

(Gems of humans radiate white, yellow, red, blue and green light and have seven qualities: (1) their color is all purifying; they dispel harms from (2) poisons, (3) spirits, (4) darkness, (5) swellings; (6) they dispel the sufferings of fevers, etc., and (7) fulfil wishes. Deva's gems have these seven qualities and also (8) accompany them everywhere, (9) are light (in weight), (10) are perfectly pure, and (11) have the ability to speak. Bodhisattva's gems have these eleven qualities and (12) enable them to see the death and rebirth of others, (13) enable them to see the time of the ultimate liberation of others, and (14) can teach in various ways according to the dispositions and aptitudes of disciples.) To the south of that city lies the mountain called Vinvya (Thunderbolt), endowed with the power of the sun. Here are found pomegranate, black pepper, longpeper, white leadwort, etc., i.e. medicines which cure cold disorders, and a forest of medicines having hot, sour, salty tastes and hot, sharp (coarse and light) powers. The medicinal roots, trunks, branches, leaves, flowers and fruits are fragrant, attractive and pleasing to behold, and wherever their scent pervades no cold disorder will arise.

To the north of the city lies the mountain called Himavata (Snow Mountain) which is endowed with the power of the moon. Here are found sandalwood, camphor, eaglewood, neem, etc., (medicines) which cure fevers, and a forest of bitter, sweet and astringent medicines having cool, blunt (and firm) powers. The medicinal roots, trunks, branches, leaves, flowers and fruits are fragrant, attractive and pleasing to behold, and wherever their scent pervades no fever will arise.

To the east of that city lies the mountain called sPos.ngad.ldan (Fragrant Mountain), upon which grows a forest of (chebulic) myrobalan. Its roots cure bone disorders, the trunks cure flesh disorders, the branches cure diseases of the channels and ligaments, the bark cures skin disorders, the leaves cure disorders of the vessel organs, the flowers cure disorders of the sense organs and the fruits cure disorders of the heart and other vital organs. At the tops (of the trees) ripen the five types of (chebulic) myrobalan which are endowed with the six tastes, the eight (natural) powers, the three post-digestive (tastes) and the seventeen secondary qualities. These cure all types of diseases and wherever the scent of these fragrant, attractive and pleasing medicines pervades, the four hundred and four diseases will not arise.

To the west of that city on the mountain called Ma.la.ya (Garlanded Mountain) grow the six superlative medicines. All diseases are healed by the five kinds of calcite, the five kinds of mineral exudate, the five kinds of medicinal water and the five kinds of hot spring which are found on this mountain.

All around the city are meadows of saffron with the wafting fragrance of incense, and all kinds of mineral medicines and salts are found in the rocks. Peacocks, cranes (*shang.shang*), parrots and other birds sing sweetly in the treetops of this forest of medicines, and on the ground dwell all kinds of animals (creatures bearing excellent medicines, e.g., elephants, bears, musk deer, etc.). Thus the region is adorned with all kinds of medicines that grow and are to be found.

In the center of the palace on a gem throne of aquamarine sat the Master of Medicine, King of Aquamarine Light, the fully endowed transcendent Conqueror who is Guide and Physician. The Master was completely surrounded by four circles of disciples, gods, sages, non-Buddhists and Buddhists. The circle of gods included the celestial physician sKyes.rguhi.bdag.po.myur.wa and Tha.skar, the divine sovereign Indra and the goddess bDud.rtsi.ma (Amritavati, who offered myrobalan to the Medicine Buddha). These and many other divine disciples were assembled there. The circle of sages included the great sage 'Son of rGyun.she' (Atreya), Mi.bzhin.hjug (Agnivesha), Mu.kyu.hdzin (Nimindhar), 'Son of hGro.bskyong', gShol.hgro.skyes, dKah.gnyis.spyod, Thang.la.hbar (Dhanvantari) and Nabs.so.skyes. These and many other sages were assembled there. The circle of non-Buddhists included Brahma, the patriarch of the Tirthikas, Mahadeva, Sri Ralpachen (Jatanika; lit. 'The One with Matted Hair'), Vishnu and gZhon.nu.gdong.drug (Kumara, the son of Mahadeva with six faces who holds a small spear and rides a peacock). These and many other non-Buddhists were assembled there. The circle of Buddhists included Arya Manjushri, the mighty Avalokiteshvara, Vajrapani, Ananda and the physician gZhon.nu (Kumara). These and many other Buddhists were assembled there. At that time each of the four circles of disciples understood the Master's words to be of the tradition of their own Master.[1]

This (particular teaching) is called the 'Tradition of Sages,'[2] for they are without faults of body, speech or mind, are upright and true, and eradicate faults in others.

This concludes the first chapter, on the basis of discussion (introduction), from *The Quintessence Tantra, the Secret Oral Tradition of the Eight Branches of the Science of Healing.*

2. The Enumeration of Topics

At that time the Master Buddha, the supreme healer and benefactor, King of Aquamarine Light, entered the meditative equipoise known as 'the Sovereign Healer who subdues the four hundred and four diseases.' As soon as he entered this absorption, from his heart were emitted in all the ten directions many hundreds of thousands of variegated rays which dispelled the mental distortions of all sentient beings in the ten directions and pacified all diseases of the three poisons arisen from ignorance. Once these had been drawn back into his heart, the emanated Master named Sage Rig.pahi.ye.she was emitted from his heart. Appearing in space before (the Buddha), he spoke these words of introduction to the circle of sages: O friends, know that he who wishes to remain free of disease, and who wishes to cure disease, should learn the oral teaching of the science of healing. He who desires long life should learn the oral (instruction) teaching of the science of healing. He who wishes to receive Dharma Teaching, wealth and happiness should learn this oral teaching on the science of healing. He who desires to liberate any being from the misery of disease and who wishes regard and respect from others should learn the oral (instruction) teaching on the science of healing.

After he had spoken these words, from the tongue of the Supreme Master, the King of Aquamarine Light, were emitted many hundreds of thousands of variegated rays in the ten directions, removing the verbal defilements of all sentient beings in all ten directions and subduing all diseases and spirits. Then, after he had drawn them back to his tongue, the emanation of the Buddha's speech, the sage Yid.las.skyes, appeared, prostrated and circumambulated (the Master). Then, in the manner of a lion, he uttered these words of request before the Master on behalf of the assembled sages: O Master, Sage Rig.pahi.ye.she, as we desire to acquire this bounty for the sake of ourselves and others, how may we learn the oral teaching of the science of healing?

At these words the mind-emanation sage gave the following reply: O Great Sages, learn the oral tradition Tantra on the science of healing. Learn the branches. Learn the principles. Learn the divisions. Learn the compilations. Learn the chapters.

At this the sage Yid.las.skyes asked: O Master, how may we learn the oral tradition Tantra on the science of healing?

The Master replied: O Great Sage, listen. Learn the Four Tantras, namely the Root Tantra, Explanatory Tantra, Oral Instruction Tantra and Final Tantra. These are known as the Four Tantras.

What are the eight branches to be learned? They are: physical disorders, disorders in children, disorders in women, diseases caused by spirits, (injuries from) weapons, poisoning, and (remedies for) aging and sterility. These are to be known as the eight branches.

What are the eleven principles to be learned? They are: (1) the principle of the synthesis of fundamentals, (2) the principle of the existence of the body (from birth to death), (3) the principle of the rise and decline of disease, (4) the principle of behavioral pattern, (5) the principle of nutrition, (6) the principle of compounding medicines, (7) the principle of surgical instruments, (8) the principle of normal health, (9) the principle of diagnosis, (10) the principle of therapeutic procedures, and (11) the principle of the function of the physician. These are known as the eleven principles.

What are the fifteen divisions to be learned? They are: (1) the division of healing (disorders of) the three humors, (2) the division of treating internal disorders, (3) the division of treating fevers, (4) the division of treating (disorders of) the upper (part of the) body, (5) the division of healing the vital and vessel organs, (6) the division of treating genital disorders, (7) the division of treating miscellaneous disorders, (8) the division of healing sores arising as a secondary condition, (9) the division of treating children, (10) the gynecology division, (11) the division of healing diseases caused by spirits, (12) the division of healing wounds caused by weapons, (13) the division of treating poisoning, (14) the division of essence-extraction (rejuvenation, etc.) and (15) the division of inducing fertility. These are known as the fifteen divisions.

What are the four compilations to be learned? They are: (1) the compilation on pulse and urine examination, (2) the compilation on medicines which subdue diseases, (3) the compilation on medicines inducing evacuation, and (4) the compilation on mild and drastic therapies. These are known as the four compilations.

What are the one hundred and fifty-six chapters to be studied? They are (as follows):

The six chapters on: (1) the basis of discussion (introduction), (2) the enumeration of topics, (3) the basis (of disease), (4) diagnosis, (5) methods of treatment, and (6) the enumeration (of metaphors). This compendium of principles is known as the Root Tantra.

The eleven principles (are contained in thirty-one chapters) in the Explanatory Tantra: (1) the summary of the Explanatory Tantra, (2) the way in which the body develops, (3) the similes (of the body), (4) anatomy, (5) physiology, (6) classifications, (7) signs of death, (8) the causes of disease, (9) immediate causes of disease, (10) the means of entry (of disease), (11) characteristics of disease, (12) classifications of disease, (13) routine behavior, (14) seasonal behavior, (15) incidental behavior, (16) diet, (17) dietary restrictions, (18) balanced intake of food, (19) the tastes (of medicines), (20) the (natural) powers of medicines, (21) methods of compounding, (22) instruments, (23) remaining healthy, (24) diagnosis, (25) examination by craft and guile, (26) four diagnostic criteria for accepting or declining to accept a patient, (27) general therapeutic techniques, (28) specific therapeutic techniques, (29) two therapeutic media, (30) direct therapeutics, (31) the doctor (i.e., his code of ethics). Three single chapters, four sets of three chapters, one set of four, one set of five and one set of six chapters, plus one summary chapter make thirty-one chapters in all.

The fifteen divisions (are contained in ninety-two chapters) in the Oral Instruction Tantra: (1) the chapter of requesting, (2) wind disorders, (3) bile disorders, (4) phlegm disorders, (5) tri-humoral disorders; [*six chapters on chronic internal disorders:*] (6) chronic abdominal and digestive disorders, (7) tumors, (8) first stage oedema, (9) second stage oedema, (10) third stage oedema, (11) consumption (tuberculosis); [*sixteen chapters on fevers:*] (12) general fevers, (13) contrary indications (bases of error), (14) the 'hill meets plain' syndrome (in which wind fans and manifests fever, but one should treat as for wind), (15) unripened fever, (16) high fever, (17) empty fevers, (18) hidden fever, (19) chronic fevers, (20) turbid fever, (21) spreading fever or scattered fever, (22) disturbed fever, (23) infectious fever, (24) poxes, (25) colic, (26) diphtheria or quinsy,[1] (27) the common cold; [*six chapters on disorders of the upper body:*] (28) head diseases, (29) eye diseases, (30) ear disorders, (31) nasal disorders, (32) mouth disorders, (33) goiters; [*eight chapters on disorders of the vital and vessel organs:*] (34) the heart, (35) the lungs, (36) the liver, (37) the spleen, (38) the kidneys, (39) the stomach, (40) the small intestine, (41) the large intestine; [*two chapters on genital disorders:*] (42) genital disorders in men and (43) in women; [*nineteen chapters on miscellaneous disorders:*] (44) hoarseness, (45) anorexia, (46) thirst, (47) hiccoughs, (48) asthma, (49) stomach cramps, (50) parasites, (51) vomiting, (52) diarrhoea, (53) constipation, (54) urinary obstruction, (55) urinary frequency (including polyuria),[2] (56) gastroenteritis, (57) gout, (58) rheumatism, (59) lymph disorders, (60) 'white nerve' (including Parkinson's disease and paralysis/polio, both viral infections of the central nervous system), (61) skin diseases, (62) minor disorders (including hangovers and *nya.log*, anterior transposition of the calf muscle); [*eight chapters on sores and ulcerations* (sometimes caused by spirits):] (63) sores and abscesses which ulcerate spontaneously because of waste blood rolled by wind to form abscesses, (64) hemorrhoids (65) erysipelas,[3] (66) Surya (metastatic cancer),[4] (67) *rmen.bu*, or lymph-caused cancer-like tumors in the form of lumps and swellings in the glands, (68) hydrocele, (69) elephantiasis,[5] (70)

anal fistula; [*three chapters on pediatrics:*] (71) treatment to
safeguard the foetus, (72) children's diseases, (73) spirit(-
caused) disorders in children; [*three chapters on gynecology:*] (74)
general gynecology, (75) specific gynecology, (76) common
gynecological disorders; [*five chapters on spirit-caused disorders:*] (77) (disorders caused by) bhuta spirits, (78) spirits
causing insanity (Skt. *apasmara*), (79) spirit-caused trance or
amnesia, (80) epilepsy (lit. 'the planets'), (81) *naga* [6] diseases;
[*five chapters on wounds and lesions:*] (82) general (treatment
of) wounds, (83) head wounds, (84) neck wounds, (85)
wounds on the trunk, (86) (wounds on) the limbs; [*three
chapters on poisoning:*] (87) compound poisons, (88) food
poisoning, (89) natural poisons (from snakes, plants, dogs,
spiders, etc.); (90) rejuvenation and essence-extraction compounds; and [*two chapters on aphrodisiacs and virilification:*]
(91) aphrodisiacs and sperm-enriching treatment, (92) inducing fertility in women.

Thus there is one single chapter, two pairs, three sets of
three, one set of four, two sets of five, two sets of six, two sets
of eight, one set of sixteen and one set of nineteen chapters.
(These together with the chapter of requesting total ninety-
two.)

The four compilations (are contained in twenty-five chapters) in the Final Tantra: [*two chapters on diagnostic media:*] (1)
pulse diagnosis, (2) urine diagnosis; [*ten chapters on pacification:*] (3) decoctions, (4) powders, (5) pills, (6) extracts, (7)
medicinal oils, (8) calcinated compounds (especially for cold
disorders), (9) concentrates,[7] (10) alcoholic medicines (for
wind disorders and phlegm-bile combinations), (11) gem
medicines,[8] (12) herbal compounds; [*seven chapters on
evacuation:*] (13) medicinal oils (for external use, e.g. for
massage), (14) purgation, (15) emesis, (16) nasal medicines,
(17) suppositories, (18) enemas, (19) channel (e.g., vein)
cleansing; and [*six chapters on (accessory) therapies:*] (20)
venesection, (21) cauterization, (22) fomentation, (23) (a)
medicinal baths (especially for stiffness of limbs, paralysis and
wind disorders) and (b) embrocation, (24) external application
(ointments), (25) spoon surgery. Thus there is one pair of
chapters, one set of ten (3-12) one set of seven (13-19) and one
set of six (20-25).

Thus, the Root Tantra has six chapters, the Explanatory Tantra has thirty-one, the Oral Instruction Tantra has ninety-two and the Final Tantra has twenty-five chapters. The Four Tantras combined contain one hundred and fifty-four chapters, plus the concluding chapter and the chapter on the type of student to whom these teachings may be imparted, making one hundred and fifty-six chapters in all. These are subsumed under the eight branches as follows: seventy chapters on the body, three chapters on children's diseases and three on gynecology, three on poisoning, five on spirits, five on wounds, one on rejuvenation (essence-extraction) and two on fertility. (The eight branches) are encompassed in the three tantras (i.e., in the Root Tantra, Explanatory Tantra and the Final Tantra).

This concludes the second chapter, on the enumeration of topics, from *The Quintessence Tantra, the Secret Oral Tradition of the Eight Branches of the Science of Healing.*

3. The Basis of Disease

Then the sage Yid.las.skyes asked the sage Rig.pahi.ye.she: O Master, Sage Rig.pahi.ye.she.la, of the four types of Tantra on the science of healing how may one learn the Root Tantra? May the Healer, King of Physicians, please explain.

At this the mind emanation Rig.pahi.ye.she replied: O Great Sage Yid.las.skyes, first I shall elucidate the combined principles of the Root Tantra. Entwined with the three roots are nine trunks, from which spread forty-seven branches. On these grow two hundred and twenty-four leaves and ripen five pristine flowers and fruits. These are said to be the summary of the Root Tantra.

To elaborate further, the three categories are the humors, bodily constituents and excretions. Their balance and imbalance respectively sustain and afflict the body.

The three humoral disorders are wind, bile and phlegm. (The five kinds of wind are) the life-supporting wind, ascending wind, pervading wind, firelike-equalizing wind and descending ("downwards-clearing") wind. (The five biles are) digestive bile, nutriment-transforming bile, accomplishing bile, sight bile and complexion-clearing bile. The five phlegms are supporting phlegm, decomposing phlegm, experiencing phlegm, satisfying phlegm and connective phlegm. (This makes) fifteen in all.

The seven bodily constituents are essential nutriment, blood, flesh, fat, bone, marrow and semen (vital fluid). The excretions are stool, urine and perspiration. Thus if these twenty-five aspects and the three factors of (1) the tastes and (2) the powers of one's diet, and (3) one's behavioral pattern are all in harmony, one will thrive and flourish. If these vary one will be afflicted.

Diseases are produced by three causes accompanied by four immediate conditions [season, spirits, food and behavioral pattern] and meet the six entrances [skin, flesh, channels, bone, vital and vessel organs] before remaining in the upper, lower, or middle body. They travel along the fifteen pathways [bone, ear, skin, heart and life channel, large intestine, blood, perspiration, eye, liver, gallbladder and small intestine, nutriment with flesh and fat, marrow and semen, stool and urine, lungs with kidneys and spleen, stomach and urinary bladder, nose and tongue] and increase according to nine factors of age [child, adult and old age]; environment [cold, hot and dry, and damp]; and season [spring, summer and autumn].

There are nine conditions which result in loss of life and twelve reaction-imbalances.

All the above factors are included in the divisions of hot and cold. Thus with regard to the sixty-three disorders to be healed, attachment, hatred and closed (-mindedness) are the three causes which in turn give rise to wind, bile and phlegm (disorders). Along with these any irregularities of the four factors of season, spirit, diet and behavioural pattern increase and decrease (the humors). (The resultant imbalance) spreads through the skin, develops in the flesh, passes through the channels, adheres to the bones, descends upon the vital organs and flows into the vessel organs.

[Seats of disease]: phlegm is based in the brain and remains in the upper body; bile is located at the level of the diaphragm and abides in the middle body, whilst wind is based at the hips and waist and abides in the lower body. The pathways of wind, bile and phlegm (disorders) are the bodily constituents, the excretions, the sense organs, and the vital and vessel organs. [Specifically the pathways of wind disorders are] the bones, ears, nerve endings, heart, life channel and large intestine. [The pathways of bile disorders are] blood, perspiration, eyes, liver, gall (-bladder) and small intestine. [The pathways of phlegm] are nutriment, flesh, fat, marrow, semen, stool, urine, nose, tongue, lungs, spleen, stomach, kidneys and urinary bladder. Aged people are "wind" people, adults are "bile" people and children (up to the age of sixteen approximately) are "phlegm" people; such are the dangers of age groups. Cold and windy places are said to be "wind" areas, whilst scorching, oppressively hot places are "bile" places, and damp, slimy places are said to be "phlegm" places.

[Rising periods of disease]: wind disorders arise in summer (monsoon), evening and around dawn. Bile (imbalances) arise in autumn, around noon and midnight, (whereas) phlegm disorders arise in spring, (early) morning and dusk.

The nine disorders which result in death are: (1) consumption of the [three factors supporting] life [i.e., of life-span, karma and merit], (2) (severe) disruption of the humors (in spite of treatment), (3) receiving treatment similar to the disease (because of earlier deceptive indications), (4) piercing of a vital organ, (5) advanced wind disorder in which the support of the life wind is lost, (6) fever beyond cure, (7) a cold disorder (beyond cure), (8) when the bodily constituents are unable to sustain the body, (9) (death due to) harm (from a spirit).

The twelve reaction imbalances are: (1) alleviating wind while transforming into bile, (2) alleviating wind while transforming into phlegm, (3) imbalance of bile after failing to alleviate wind, (4) imbalance of phlegm after ailing to alleviate wind, (5) alleviating bile while transforming into wind, (6) alleviating bile while transforming into phlegm, (7) imbalance of wind while failing to alleviate bile, (8) imbalance of phlegm while failing to alleviate bile, (9) alleviating phlegm while transforming into wind, (10) alleviating phlegm while transforming into bile, (11) imbalance of wind while failing to alleviate phlegm, (12) imbalance of bile while failing to alleviate phlegm.

Wind and phlegm disorders are (classified as) cold and (likened to) water. Blood and bile are asserted to be hot and are likened to fire. Parasites and lymph disorders are both common to hot and cold disorders. Thus from the eighty-eight categories above one will understand all the basic aspects of diseases.

Thus it was said. This concludes the third chapter, on the basis of disease, from *The Quintessence Tantra, the Secret Oral Tradition of the Eight Branches of the Science of Healing*.

4. Diagnosis and Symptoms

Then the sage Rig.pahi.ye.she said these words: O Great Sage, listen. Disease may be fully understood from visual (examination), palpation and questioning.

Visual examination entails checking the tongue and urine. This diagnosis involves understanding a visual object. Contact of the fingers with the pulse is the source of signals communicated (from within the body), and such diagnosis entails understanding of (these) objects of analysis. One questions the patient verbally regarding the conditions which precipitated (the disorder), his symptoms and his diet. This [mode of] diagnosis involves hearing and understanding (the patient's) voice.

In wind (disorders) the tongue will be red, dry and rough, (whilst) in a bile disorder the tongue will be covered by a thick, pale yellow coating of phlegm. In a phlegm disorder the tongue will have a pale, thick coating of phlegm and be dull, smooth and moist.

Urine in wind disorders looks like water and has large bubbles. In a bile disorder the urine is reddish yellow and malodorous, with much steam. Urine (reflecting a) phlegm disorder is whitish with little odor or steam.

The wind pulse is floating, empty and halting. The bile pulse has a rapid, prominent, taut beat, whilst the phlegm pulse is sunken, weak and ponderous.

With regard to questioning, (the immediate) causes of a wind disorder are light, coarse diet and behavioral patterns (e.g., tea, pork, goat's meat and fasting). The symptoms will include yawning, trembling, stretching, shivering, shifting and uncertain pain in the hips, waist-bones and all joints, dry heaves, dullness of the sense organs, mental instability and hunger pains. Oily and nutritious foods are certain to be beneficial (as well as relaxing in warm, dim surroundings with anyone you feel at ease with, enjoying soothing conversation, sweet music, etc.). Avoid large lakes and oceans, places where animals are slaughtered, abysses, etc., and avoid climbing trees, etc.

Sharp, hot food and behavioral factors [contribute to bile disorders], e.g., matured wines, vinegar, mutton fat, sitting in hot sun or other very hot places, and sudden or strenuous physical activity. [The symptoms are] bitter taste in the mouth, headaches, surface or flesh fever, pain in the upper body and post-digestive pain. Cool-powered food and behavioral pattern are beneficial [for bile cases, e.g., curd, whey, beef or goat meat, and sitting in a cool, breezy place].

[Phlegm disorders are developed by] heavy, oily food and behavioral pattern (e.g., sitting and sleeping on grass and earth). [The symptoms are] anorexia, difficulty in digesting food, vomiting, loss of sense of taste, distention (and heaviness) of the stomach, belching, heaviness of body and mind, coldness both externally and internally, and discomfort after eating. (To remedy) phlegm disorders warm food and behavioral pattern are favorable (such as old wine, ginger, mutton, ginger decoction, pomegranate, cinnamon, longpeper, wearing warm clothes, and sitting near a fire or in the sun).

Thus, by means of these thirty-eight diagnostic methods one can unerringly and faultlessly ascertain (the nature) of all disease.

Thus it was said. This concludes the fourth chapter, on diagnosis and symptoms, from *The Quintessence Tantra, the Secret Oral Tradition of the Eight Branches of the Science of Healing.*

5. Methods of Treatment

Then the sage Rig.pahi.ye.she spoke these words: O Great Sage, listen! The remedies for healing disease are fourfold: diet, behavioral pattern, medicine and accessory therapy.

DIET

(Firstly) the recommended diet for wind disorders (includes) meat of horse, donkey and marmot, one-year-old (dried) meat, human flesh,[1] seed oil, one-year-old butter, raw cane sugar, garlic, onion, milk, grain beer with angelica root and *Polygonatum cirrifolium,* wine of cane sugar and bone wine.

The (curative) foods recommended for bile disorders are curd and whey made from cow's or goat's milk, fresh butter, game meat (e.g., deer), goat meat, fresh meat of she-yak-calf or of ox-dzo cross, fresh grain porridge, *kyabs* [a type of dandelion] stew, dandelion stew (or grey dandelion stew), and warm water, cool (spring) water or cold boiled water.

The diet to be followed in phlegm disorders consists of mutton, wild yak meat, meat of carnivorous animals and fish, honey, stored grain grown in a dry area, cooked doughballs, curd and whey from she-yak's milk, thick (old) wine, and (hot) boiled water.

BEHAVIORAL PATTERN

The wind (patient) should stay in a warm place and in pleasant company. The bile (patient) should stay in a cool place and rest, whilst phlegm cases should take exercise and stay in warm places.

MEDICINES

[Medicines for wind disorders] should be sweet [e.g., cane sugar]; sour [e.g., wine, vinegar, pomegranate]; salty [e.g., lake salt]; and with oily [e.g., eaglewood tree], heavy [e.g., black salt] and smooth [e.g., Indian Salamin] powers.

Bile medicines should be sweet [e.g., raisin]; bitter [e.g., bitter cucumber]; astringent [e.g., white sandalwood]; and with cool [e.g., camphor], fluid [e.g., Cassia pods] and blunt [e.g., bamboo concretion] powers.

[Medicines for] phlegm disorders should be hot (tasting) [e.g., black pepper]; sour [e.g., pomegranate]; astringent [e.g., beleric myrobalan]; and with sharp [e.g., rock salt], coarse [e.g., berries of sea buckthorn] and light [e.g., white leadwort] powers.

With (these) tastes and powers are combined the two (techniques of) pacification and evacuation.

For the pacification of wind disorders (the following are used): soup [e.g., of sheep's knee-bone, of the four essences - meat, grain beer, cane sugar and butter, or of one-year-old (finely-ground) sheep's head] or medicinal butters [e.g., of nutmeg, garlic or the three myrobalan fruits, or of the five roots, including small caltrops, *Angelica* sp., and black aconite].

Bile disorders are pacified in reliance upon decoctions [e.g., decoctions of *Iris germanica,* heart-leaved moonseed, chiretta and the three (myrobalan) fruits] and powders [e.g., of camphor, white sandalwood, saffron or bamboo concretion as principal ingredients].

Phlegm disorders [are pacified] by compounds (in the form of) pills [principally of black aconite or of various salts] and calcinated powders (*tres.sam*) e.g., of pomegranate, white flower of *Rhododendron anthopogonoides, rgod.ma.kha* [a pungent medicinal mixture, e.g., the 'sixfold compound of

Indian beech'], or of calcinated salts or calcinated calcite.

Evacuation of wind disorders entails (the use of) suppositories, bile disorders (require) purgation and in phlegm cases emesis (is induced).

Suppositories consist of: (1) *sle.hjam* (mild suppository), (2) *btru.hjam* (suppository, following insertion of which the patient's feet are clapped together to distribute the'medicine through the tract), and (3) *bkru.ma.slen* (suppository similar to the previous one and which is distributed by shaking the patient's legs).

Purgation (of bile disorders) is of general, specific, drastic and mild types. Emesis is applied in strong (with the patient in squatting position) and mild ways.

ACCESSORY THERAPIES

Treatment by accessory therapy: accessory therapies (for wind) consist of massage with an embrocation of sesame oil and Turkestani moxa cauterization (a type of hot poultice using cloth containing fennel, dipped in hot oil and applied, e.g., to four points on the head).

Accessory therapies [used in bile disorders] include sudorifics, venesection and devices (such as) cold water bottle fomentation. [Phlegm accessory therapy] entails fomentation [e.g., with heated salts applied to the abdomen] and cauterization (e.g., on the joints, with metal instruments or standard moxa).

Thus, by relying upon these ninety-eight healing techniques with care, respect and diligence one will be quickly freed from the mire of disease.

Thus it was said. This concludes the fifth chapter, on healing techniques, from *The Quintessence Tantra, the Secret Oral Tradition of the Eight Branches of the Science of Healing.*

6. The Enumeration of Metaphors

Then again the sage Rig.pahi.ye.she spoke these words:

O Great Sage, listen! Around the (three) roots of the natural state of the body, diagnosis, and treatment are entwined the nine trunks of: the normally functioning body, the malfunctioning body, visual examination, palpation, questioning, diet, behavioral pattern, medicine, and accessory therapy.

The forty-seven branches (on the trunks) are: on the (first trunk of the) healthy body (1) the humors, (2) the bodily constituents, and (3) the excretions; on the (second trunk of the) diseased body (4) the causes, (5) immediate causes, (6) the entrances, (7) locations, (8) pathways, (9) time of arisal, (10) (fatal) result, (11) side effects, and (12) categories (hot and cold).

(On the third trunk of) visual examination (13) the tongue and (14) urine; (on the fourth trunk) the three (types of) pulse ((15) wind, (16) bile and (17) phlegm); (on the fifth trunk of) questioning (are the) three (branches) of (18) precipitating conditions, (19) symptoms, and (20) (living and eating) habits.

(On the sixth trunk of) diet are the six branches of food and drink (consisting of) (21 & 22) recommended foods and beverages (for wind patients), (23 & 24) recommended foods and beverages (for bile patients) and (25 & 26) foods and beverages (for phlegm patients).

(On the seventh trunk) are the three (branches of) living

habits for those with (27) wind, (28) bile, and (29) phlegm disorders.

(On the eighth trunk of) medicine are three pairs of branches, i.e. both tastes and powers of (30 & 31) wind medicines, (32 & 33) bile medicines, and (34 & 35) phlegm medicines. The six pacification techniques (consist of) both (36) soups and (37) medicinal oils (for wind); (38) decoctions (for bile) and (39) powders (for bile); (40) pills and (41) (calcinated) powders (for phlegm). The three types of evacuation (are) (42) (use of) suppositories (for wind), (43) purgation (for bile), and (44) emesis (for phlegm).

(On the ninth trunk are) the three (branches of) accessory therapy for (45) wind (oil massage and Turkestani moxa), (46) bile (sudorifics, venesection and cold fomentation), and (47) phlegm (hot fomentation and moxabustion).

There are twenty-five leaves on the first (trunk of good health), sixty-three leaves on the (second) summarized pathology trunk, six leaves on the visual examination trunk, three leaves (on the trunk) of pulses to be felt and twenty-nine (on the trunk) of questioning.

(On the) diet (trunk) are fourteen leaves of diet to be followed in wind disorders, twelve for bile and nine for phlegm-oriented foods and drinks. On the behavioral pattern trunk are six leaves and on the medicines trunk are nine leaves for taste, nine for the powers, three for soups, five for the types of medicinal oil, four decoctions, four powders, two types of pill, five calcinated powders (*bhasmas*), nine unsurpassed therapies (emesis, etc.) and seven classes of accessory therapy. Thus there are eighty-eight leaves for the basis of disease (pathology), thirty-eight for diagnosis and ninety-eight healing techniques making a sum total of two hundred and twenty-four.

On the first trunk blossom the flowers of good health and long life and ripen the three fruits of Dharma, affluence and happiness (these are attained by the physician). This Root Tantra in which is compiled the essence-enumeration (of the features of the science of healing) illustrated with similes can be applied by those of sharp intellect but will not be comprehended by persons with dull minds. (The latter) should study more elaborate and detailed texts.

Having thus spoken, the sage Rig.pahi.ye.she dissolved back into the heart of the Sovereign Healer. This concludes the sixth chapter and the Root Tantra of *The Quintessence Tantra, the Secret Oral Tradition of the Eight Branches of the Science of Healing.*

PART II

THE EXPLANATORY TANTRA

1. The Summary of the Explanatory Tantra

Then the Master, the fully endowed transcendent Conqueror and Physician, King of Aquamarine Light, arose from that absorption and entered the (meditative) equipoise of healing called the 'Lion of Speech.' As soon as he entered into equipoise, from the crown of his head hundreds of thousands of variegated rays were emitted in the ten directions, removing the physical defilements of all living beings in all ten directions, and, having pacified all diseases of wind, bile and phlegm, they were collected back to the crown of his head. Then the emanated Master, the sage called Rig.pahi.ye.she, was projected from his body and appeared in space before him.

The emanation from the (Buddha's) speech, called Sage Yid.las.skyes, prostrated to the Master, circumambulated him and said these words: O Master, Sage Rig.pahi.ye.she, thus you have expounded the condensed meaning of the Root Tantra. How may one learn the Explanatory Tantra? May the Healer, King of Physicians, please explain.

At this request the emanation from the Body (of the Buddha), the sage Rig.pahi.ye.she, said these words: O Great Sage Yid.las.skyes, secondly, (with regard) to learning the Explanatory Tantra to sustain health, treat disease and ensure long life, Dharma, wealth and happiness in regard to the body of humans who are chief among the six (types of) being, I shall summarize the main points of the science of healing.

The four factors are said to be (1) the object to be healed, (2) the healing agent, (3) the method of healing, and (4) the healer.

The object to be healed will be taught first. (i) For what purpose is the body healed? What is to be healed? (ii) The diseases arising from it. The remedies that heal disease are (iii) behavioral pattern, (iv) diet, (v) medicine and (vi) accessory therapy, and how they heal disease is by (vii) maintaining health, promoting longevity and redressing physical imbalances. To this end are expounded the three (sections of) (viii) methods of diagnosis, (ix) the application of healing methods (following identification of the disease), (x) which therapeutic media are used to treat (the disorder) and (xi) (the healer) by whom the therapies are applied.

Thus, O healer, the eleven branches on the four roots are the synthesis of the Explanatory Tantra.

This concludes the first chapter, showing the summary of the Explanatory Tantra, from *The Quintessence Tantra, the Secret Oral Tradition of the Eight Branches of the Science of Healing.*

2. The Way in Which the Body Is Formed

Then the sage Yid.las.skyes asked the Master, Sage Rig.pahi.ye.she: O Master, Sage Rig.pahi.ye.she, how should one study the principles of the formation of the body? May the Healer, King of Physicians, please explain.

At this the Master replied: O Great Sage, listen. Firstly, the teaching on the body formed [of five elements] with regard to which healing takes place, is explained in seven [divisions]: (1) the manner of formation (chapter two), (2) similes (chapter three), (3) anatomy (chapter four), (4) physiology (chapter five), (5) classifications and (6) actions (chapter six), and (7) signs of death (chapter seven).

The first of these, the teaching on the way in which the body is formed, is threefold: (a) the causes of formation, (b) conditions which assist development, and (c) signs of birth.

THE CAUSES OF FORMATION

First, the causes of formation in the womb are non-defective sperm and blood of the father and mother, the consciousness impelled by karma (actions) and by the afflictive emotions and the assembled five elements. This resembles, for example, the arisal of fire from friction (between pieces of) wood.

By virtue of many of the (following) defects, the seed (of the embryo) will not be able (to come into being). Semen and blood affected by a wind imbalance will become coarse, dark and astringent. A bile imbalance will render them sour, yellow and malodorous, whilst phlegm will turn them grey, adhesive, sweet and cool. Disordered blood will cause the semen and blood to putrefy, whilst a combined phlegm-wind imbalance will fragment them. Disordered blood and bile render them pus-like, whereas they become 'knotted' by a combined phlegm-bile imbalance. A dual wind and bile imbalance dry the semen and blood, whilst a tri-humoral disorder causes them to become like stool and urine.

If the karm(ic factors) are not assembled the consciousness will not enter [the union of semen and blood]. Without the earth element, formation cannot take place, whereas without the water element the combining [of semen and blood] cannot occur. Without the fire element there will be no maturation and without the wind element no growth. (Lastly) the absence of the space element will not afford room for growth.

In the case of non-defective (vital fluids) which cause conception, the semen will be white, heavy, sweet and abundant whereas the blood will resemble [the sap of the Butea gum tree] or rabbit's blood, and (clothes can easily) be washed clean of it.

In a woman between the ages of twelve and fifty, each month blood accumulates from the essential nutriment. For three days (each time) this dark, odorless blood is expelled by the downwards voiding wind through the door of the womb and it descends through two large channels (uterine tubes). In a woman having her period the noticeable signs of her desire for a man are languor, facial ugliness (e.g. flaccidity) and quivering of the breasts, hips, throat, eyes and sides (of the body).

Once the womb has opened and up until the twelfth day (after the menstrual period) conception can occur. During the first three days (of menstruation) and on the eleventh (day) a boy will not be conceived. On the first, third, fifth, seventh and ninth (of the twelve days) a boy will be conceived and on the second, fourth, sixth and eighth days a girl will be conceived. Like the closing of the lotus after sunset, once twelve days have passed the womb does not receive semen. If the semen predominates a boy will be born and if the blood predominates a girl will be born. If the ratios are equal the result will be a neuter (or hermaphrodite) and if (the mixture) is divided [by wind] twins will be born. Birth with non-human form or with physical deformities comes about through harmful impurities (of wind, etc.).

Upon conception the semen is held in the womb and once (the woman's) desire has been satisfied her body becomes languid and heavy.

From the father's semen the bones, brain and spinal cord are produced whereas from the blood of the mother the flesh, blood and vital and vessel organs are produced. The sense consciousnesses arise from the mind of [the fetus] itself whilst from the earth element are produced the flesh, bones, nose sense base and smell. From the water element the blood, tongue sense base, taste and moisture are formed, whilst from the fire element are produced heat, clear complexion, the eye sense base and form. The wind element produces the breath, skin and objects of touch whereas the orifices, ear sense base and sound arise from the space element. According to familiarization (from previous lives) one engages in actions and appearances arise (from birth), and by the interrelationship and aggregation of causes and conditions the body is formed.

CONDITIONS WHICH ASSIST DEVELOPMENT

The instruction on the mode of development following conception is as follows: the cause of development of the fetus is the placenta. On the right and left sides of the uterus are two channels connecting the nucleus with the ovaries which are relied upon for nourishment. Thus by the nourishment from the mother's food (the fetus) is fully developed stage by stage in the womb, just as fields are irrigated by channels from the reservoir. Moreover for thirty-eight weeks (the fetus) undergoes transformation by the wind and is developed in nine months.

During the first week of the first month the mixture of sperm and blood resembles milk which has curdled. During the second week it (thickens) and lengthens, and in the third week it takes on the appearance of curd. For those desiring a boy certain methods may be used at this time but they should be applied before the sex (of the embryo) is determined. The force

50   *Quintessence Tantras of Tibetan Medicine*

of the (following) methods will prevail even over the karma (of the fetus). At this time of the 'victory' (*rgyal*) star one should make a statue of a boy (four fingerbreadths high from 'male iron' alone, or) from various types of well-beaten iron (i.e. three or five types—an uneven number) and heat it over a coal fire until it discolors. This alloy will cause hissing when placed in cow's milk as many times as the number (of types of iron used) and then two palmfuls of the liquid should be given (to the mother-to-be). She should also drink the 'nutrient of sun and moon' (*lha.tsher.dmar.po* and sterilized mercury). The omens of tying and fastening should also be applied. ('Tying' refers to tying around the woman's waist a three-stranded thread woven from the shoulder wool of one, three or five sheep—any odd number. 'Fastening' involves wrapping the statue in ram's skin and fastening it in an upright position against the womb.)

For eight months (the pregnant woman) should avoid intercourse, violent activity, not sleeping at night, sleeping in the daytime, strongly contracting (the abdominal muscles), hot, sharp and heavy (foods), constipating foods, enemas, [emetics] and venesection (blood-letting). Why? (Because these) will cause the fetus to die, be aborted or (by force of wind) to dry up in the womb.

In the fourth week (the embryo) will be (either) rounded, oval or elongated according to whether it will gradually transform into a boy, girl or neuter (or hermaphrodite) (respectively). The signs (of this stage of pregnancy) are heaviness in the hips, flaccidity, loss of appetite, yawning, stretching, lethargy, enlargement of the breasts, a liking for sour (foods), and a heartfelt desire for various kinds of food (due to the influence of the being in her womb). If these desires are obstructed the fetus will die or take on an unpleasant form. Therefore although it may be harmful, for the sake (of both mother and child) a little (of the desired food should be mixed with wholesome food) and given (to the mother).

During the second month, in the fifth week the navel first forms on the body of the fetus and in the sixth week, in dependence upon the navel, the life channel is formed [and reaches a height of sixteen fingerbreadths]. In the seventh week the eye sense base takes shape, whilst in dependence upon it the shape of the head appears in the eighth week.

During the ninth week the shape of the body (and in particular) the upper and lower trunk are formed, whilst during the third month in the tenth week the protrusions of the two shoulders and two hips appear. In the eleventh week the nine orifices are formed and in the twelfth the five vital organs take shape. During the thirteenth week the six vessel (organs) are formed and during the fourth month in the fourteenth week the upper arms and thighs take shape. In the fifteenth week the forearms and calves protrude whereas in the sixteenth the twenty digits appear.

Then during the seventeenth week all the channels which connect the outer and inner (body) are formed. During the fifth month, in the eighteenth week the flesh and fat are formed and in the nineteenth week the ligaments and tendons take shape. The bones and marrow are formed during the twentieth week and in the twenty-first week the body is encased by the skin.

Then during the sixth month, in the twenty-second week the nine orifices fully open, whilst in the twenty-third week the hair, body hair and nails are produced. In the twenty-fourth week the vital and vessel organs are clearly matured and at that time (the fetus) begins to recognize pleasure and pain. During the twenty-fifth week the movement of wind (e.g., breath) through the orifices occurs and in the twenty-sixth week the faculty of memory becomes (extremely) clear (and the fetus can even recall previous lives).

Then in the seventh month from the twenty-seventh to thirtieth weeks all (parts of the body) reach a clear state of completion, whilst during the eighth month from the thirty-first week to the thirty-fifth week all (parts) increase in size and the mother and child alternate in appearance. In the ninth month, from the thirty-sixth week onwards the child directly recognizes (his situation) with unhappiness and disgust and in the thirty-seventh week a recognition arises (that he wishes to experience something) opposite (to his present conditions. If a boy he feels attachment for his mother and animosity toward his father.)

SIGNS OF BIRTH

In the thirty-eighth week the child turns over and emerges from the womb. However the birth will be delayed if: (i) the fetus cannot develop owing to the mother's losing blood during pregnancy, (ii) the womb expands (due to nutritious diet) and makes the birth difficult when the period of gestation is completed, or (iii) the descending wind blocks the vagina at this time.

When nine months have passed and the time of birth is nigh a boy will be born if the (mother's) right side is firm, if the right side of the womb is higher, if her body feels light, if she sees men in her dreams, or if the right breast gives milk first. The signs that a girl will be born are if the mother desires contact with a man, if she delights in singing, dancing, (wearing) ornaments, or if signs opposite to the above appear (e.g. if the left side of the womb is higher). If these (opposite) signs combine a neuter (or hermaphrodite) will be born and if the center of the womb is low and the two sides are high twins will be born.

Then the signs that the birth is imminent are lassitude, relaxing of the uterus, heaviness in the lower body, pain in the pelvic region and waist, and (itching and) stabbing pains in the genitals and lower abdomen. Then the vulva opens, much urine (is passed) and pain arises uncontrollably. The woman in labor should have attendants on hand and thus the pain that will seemingly deprive her of life will be greatly relieved, and finally removed (by nutritious food).

This concludes the second chapter, showing the way in which the body is formed, from *The Quintessence Tantra, the Secret Oral Tradition of the Eight Branches of the Science of Healing.*

3. Similes of the Body

Then the sage Rig.pahi.ye.she spoke these words: O Great Sage, listen. The exposition of the structure of the aggregates by similes (on the lines of the palace of a Universal Monarch (Cakra King) is as follows:)

The two hip bones are like the foundation for the walls. The spine is like a pile of gold coins and the life-channel is like a pillar of agate (*mchhong*).[1] The square sternum (breast-bone) is like the supporting beam whilst the twenty-four ribs closely resemble the cross-beams. The costal cartilages are like (projecting) brackets. The channels and ligaments are like a network of roof-laths (struts), whilst the flesh and skin are like the plaster. The two clavicles are like the outside parapet of the mansion whereas the scapulas are like a moulding. The top of the head is like a dome whilst the five sense-doors (eyes, etc.) are like windows. The cranium is like an expansive fitted roof whereas the crown aperture is like a chimney. The right and left ears are like a garuda's wings whilst the nostrils are like an exquisite crown ornament. The hair on man or woman is like tiles, and the two arms are like pendent banners.

The upper and lower trunk are like upper and lower courtyards whilst the diaphragm is like a drawn curtain. The heart is like a king seated on his throne. The five posterior lobes are like the innermost ministers (of the king) and the five anterior lobes are like his princes. The liver and spleen are like the major and minor queens (respectively) whereas the kidneys are like the (outer) ministers or like mighty supporting beamlike strongmen. The seminal vesicle is like the treasury whilst the stomach is like the cooking pot (in which the ingredients) are stirred. The small and large intestines are like the attendants of the queen and the gall bladder is like a bag of extra ingredients. The urinary bladder is like a filled pitcher whilst the urinary duct and rectum are like water (outflow) pipes. The two legs are like the platform that enables one to dismount a horse, whereas the delicate vital parts of the body are like (those who act with the) authority granted by the king.

Thus it was said. This concludes the third chapter, showing the similes of the body, from *The Quintessence Tantra, the Secret Oral Tradition of the Eight Branches of the Science of Healing.*

4. Anatomy

Then the sage Rig.pahi.ye.she spoke these words: O Great Sage, listen. The exposition of the anatomy of the body has four aspects: (a) the anatomical presentation of the quantities of the bodily constituents; (b) the anatomical presentation of the circulatory system; (c) the anatomical presentation of the delicate, vital points; and (d) the anatomical presentation of the pathways and orifices.

THE QUANTITIES OF THE BODILY CONSTITUENTS

The amount of wind (in the body) would fill the urinary bladder whilst the quantity of bile would fill the scrotum.[1] The quantity of phlegm would fill three cupped handfuls and the amounts of blood and stool would each fill seven cupped handfuls. The amounts of urine and lymph would each fill four cupped handfuls whereas the quantities of body oil and fat would each fill two cupped handfuls. The quantities of nutritive essence and semen would each fill a single handful whilst the amount of brain would fill a single cupped handful. The quantity of flesh is five hundred fist-sizes with the (total) addition of twenty fist-sizes for the thighs and breasts of women and (the amount of menstrual blood in women would fill two cupped handfuls).

The quantity of bones includes twenty-three types. The spinal column consists of twenty-eight vertebrae whilst the ribs number twenty-four. There are thirty-two teeth, three hundred and sixty fractional bones, twelve types of major joints, two hundred and ten minor joints, sixteen (large) ligaments (behind the knees, in the ankles, in the ante cubital fossae and in the wrists, two adjacent to the spine, two inside the spine, two in the throat and two in the neck) and nine hundred tendons.

There are twenty-one thousand hairs (on the head) and (thirty-five) million hair-pores [seven million above the neck, three million five-hundred thousand on each limb and fourteen million on the rest of the body].

Also there are five vital organs, six vessel organs and nine orifices.

The ideal size of the (human) body on earth is six feet square (four cubits) (from head to toe and from fingertips to fingertips of outstretched arms), whereas a malformed body is three and a half of its own forearmspan square.

THE CIRCULATORY SYSTEM

The anatomical presentation of the circulatory system (concerns) the four types of channel: (1) the channels of formation, (2) the channels of existence, (3) the connecting channels, and (4) the life channels. [The channels, wind-energies and drops are the basis of the mind.]

The Channels of Formation
There are three channels of formation extending from the navel (e.g. of the fetus).

One of these channels (the neural tube) ascends and thereby the brain is formed. Closed-mindedness relies upon and is located in the brain, and it gives rise to phlegm (disorders) which are situated in the upper body. The (second) channel (the hepatic artery) runs through the middle (body) and conveys (the nutriment to the liver. Thence it branches off to the tenth vertebra in reliance upon which point) it forms the (black) life channel. Anger arises in reliance upon the life channel and blood, and abides in them. Bile (disorders) are produced (from anger) and are located in the middle body.

The (third) channel descends and from it are formed the genitals. In these abides attachment, which in turn produces wind, which resides (with its causes, immediate conditions and effects) in the lower body.

The Channels of Existence

The channels of existence are of four types, the first of which enables the sense faculties (to apprehend) their (respective) objects. It is situated in the brain and is surrounded by five hundred minor channels. The (second) channel of existence, at the heart, clarifies the faculty of memory and is also surrounded by five hundred minor channels. The (third) channel of existence, at the navel, forms the physical aggregates and it is surrounded by five hundred minor channels. The (fourth) channel of existence at the genitals promotes the family lineage and is surrounded by five hundred minor channels.

(These channels connect) the upper, lower, and side part of the body and hold together all the (parts, humors, constituents, excretions, etc, of the) body.

The Connecting Channels

There are two connecting channels—light and dark. From the trunk-like vital channel the twenty-four great flesh- and blood-increasing channels extend upwards in the manner of branches. Eight great hidden channels (also branch off in the same way and) connect with the vital and vessel organs, whilst sixteen visible channels connect with the limbs externally. From these (last twenty-four visible and hidden channels) branch off seventy-seven channels used for blood-letting.

There are one hundred and twelve vital channels (to which) damage [is fatal] and one hundred and eighty-nine minor channels which combine with them. These are connected to the outside (of the body) by one hundred and twenty channels, to the inside (of the body) by (another) one hundred and twenty channels and by a (further) one hundred and twenty channels to the intermediate areas (bone, marrow) of the body. From those [the one hundred and eighty-nine minor channels] branch off a further three hundred and sixty subsidiary channels from which (in turn) spread (another) seven hundred subsidiary channels. The latter connect with (an even denser) network of minor channels throughout the body.

There are nineteen (small) ligaments, with their respective functions, which descend like roots from the great ocean of channels at the brain. Thirteen hidden tendons hang down like tassels and connect internally with the vital and vessel organs, whilst six visible tendons connect externally with the limbs. From these (six) branch off sixteen minor ligaments (as well as other smaller ones).

The Life Channels
The human organism has three types of life channel. The first pervades the head and entire body. The second accompanies the respiration and the third one is like the life-base and extends (throughout the body). Since (these three) channels connect the outer and inner body by (providing) passageways for the wind and blood (and thus enable) the body to develop and thrive, and because the life-force abides in them, they are called the life channels.

THE VULNERABLE POINTS

The seven vital, vulnerable points are the flesh, fat, bones, tendons, vital and vessel organs, and channels. Injury to the flesh results in swelling whilst injury to the bones causes great pain. Injury to the tendons produces deformity, whereas injury to the channels, fat, vital and vessel organs results in loss of life. These are called vulnerable points because (injury to them) is so difficult to heal that death (may result).

There are forty-five vulnerable points of flesh, eight of fat, thirty-two of bone, fourteen of the tendons, thirteen of the vital and vessel organs, and one hundred and ninety vital channels. Of these sixty-two are in the head, thirty-three in the neck, ninety-five in the upper and lower trunk, and one hundred and twelve are in the four limbs. Thus the total number of vulnerable points is said to be three hundred and two, of which ninety-six are extremely vital. If (the latter) are pierced the life will be lost and even (if the doctor) is skilled no cure (will be possible).

The medium vital points are said to number forty-nine and can be healed by a skilled doctor. Although the remainder (one hundred and fifty-seven) are indicated as vulnerable, they are not said to be vital, for all of them can be healed.

THE PATHWAYS AND ORIFICES

The structure of the pathways and orifices is twofold: internal and external. The internal orifices are threefold: the life force, the constituents and excretions. There are thirteen pathways for liquids and solids: (1) the great central life channel which is the pathway of the wind energy, (2) the pathway of nutriment from the stomach to the liver, (3) the pathway of blood from the liver to the flesh, (4) the pathway of flesh from the blood to the fat, (5) the pathway of fat from flesh to bone, (6) the pathway of bone from fat to marrow, (7) the pathway of marrow from bone to white and red vital fluids, (8)the pathway of red and white vital fluids from marrow to seminal vesicle, (9) the pathway of stool from stomach to anus, (10) the pathway of urine from stomach to urinary bladder, (11) the pores as the pathway of perspiration, (12) the pathway of food, and (13) the trachea.

There are seven external openings in the head and two in the genital area. Women have the extra openings of the vagina and the two breasts.

The shapes (of the pathways) are round, broad, thin and long, and they are (inter-) connected and spreading like the veins on the back of a leaf. The nutriment (energy) (of each bodily constituent) readily increases upon entering the pathways and through indulgence in inappropriate diet or behaviour (one humor may increase and disturb the other two). Thus the pathways are impaired and disease arises. [At this time the bodily constituents and excretions] increase or block (the pathways and overflow from their individual seats and) enter (the wrong channels of) other (constituents, etc.). (Thus each) disturbs (the next one in turn. When the pathways remain) clear and unimpaired one will be at ease.

Thus it was said. This concludes the fourth chapter, presenting the anatomy of the body, from *The Quintessence Tantra, the Secret Oral Tradition of the Eight Branches of the Science of Healing.*

5. Physiology

Then the sage Rig.pahi.ye.she spoke these words: O Great Sage, listen. The characteristics of the body (physiology) are twofold: the spheres which are the objects of harm, and the humors which are the harmers. Owing to the inter-dependence of each of the individual humors, bodily constituents and excretions, the body arises, endures and disintegrates; and because the aggregates so formed are the root of this process they are called 'the body.'

SPHERES OF THE OBJECTS OF HARM

Firstly, the spheres of the objects of harm are classified as: (1) the digestive heat, (2) its method of transforming, and (3) the time of completion of its results.

The (actual) objects of harm are classified as the bodily constituents and the excretions. The seven bodily constituents are said to be the nutriment, blood, flesh, fat, bone, marrow and vital fluid. The excretions are stool, urine and perspiration, etc. and are also (objects of harm).

The nutriment develops the objects of harm (especially blood), the blood 'moistens' the body and sustains life, the flesh covers the body, the fat 'lubricates' it, the bones provide support, the marrow transforms into essential nutriments, and the vital fluid contributes (to conception in) the womb. The stool and urine support (other) decomposing (matter above them) and are expelled (from the body). The perspiration keeps the skin supple and the pores firm.

The Digestive Heat

The (digestive) heat is the basis of the digestive (process) and refers to the digestive bile. It supplies heat to the humors, bodily constituents and excretions, (ensures) good health, energy, radiance of complexion, (long) life, and it increases the heat and strength of the bodily constituents. It [separates nutriment and waste], conveys the wastes from the area of digestion and bars undigested food from entering the pathway of digested food. If the digestive heat is strong the digested material moves downwards after digestion, (but if it is) weak the food is passed undigested. The digestive heat causes the food to increase the bodily constituents, the complexion and strength of the body. (However) if the food is not digested the nutriment, etc. will not increase. Therefore if one protects the digestive heat by endeavoring to partake of warm (-powered) and light food, drink and behavioral pattern, the strength and life of the body will be preserved.

Digestion

The manner in which the digestive heat digests the food (is as follows): the life [-sustaining] wind conveys the food and drink to the stomach where the drink breaks up (the material) and the oil content softens it. The firelike equalizing wind fans the digestive bile (in a manner which) resembles boiling medicine in the stomach. First the decomposing phlegm [earth and water] breaks down whatever food and drink of the six tastes (have been consumed). (In the process the food and drink) become sweet [earth and water] and foamy, and the phlegm increases. In the intermediate phase the digestive bile [fire and earth] digests [the contents of the stomach] making them extremely hot and sour [fire and earth] whilst the bile increases. Finally the firelike equalizing wind [water and wind] separates the nutriment and wastes, giving way to bitter [water and wind] taste (in the stomach) and thereby wind increases.

The qualities of the five elements of the food develop the five elements of the body. The (mode) of transformation after digested food has been separated into nutriment and waste products (is as follows): The wastes are divided into solid and fluid wastes in the small intestine; the solids become stool and the fluids become urine. The nutriment is ripened by the heat of each of the bodily constituents (and) from the stomach it is conveyed to the nine nutriment-bearing channels through the liver pathway. In the liver it becomes blood and thence turns into flesh and in turn fat, bone and marrow, and finally it transforms into vital fluid.

With regard to the wastes of these (constituents), the waste product of the (initial) nutriment becomes the (decomposing) phlegm of the stomach; (the waste from the blood becomes) the bile in the gall bladder; (the waste from the flesh turns into) the impurities emitted from the orifices (such as from the ears, eyes, etc.); (the waste from the fat becomes) the oil (component of the body); (the waste from the bones) becomes teeth, nails and hair (on the body); (whilst the waste from the marrow becomes) (skin), stool and grease component. (Finally) the waste product of the vital fluid sustains the semen. The bodily constituent of vital fluid has the supreme quintessential vital essence and although it abides in the heart (its vitality) pervades the whole body. It is the foundation of life and provides bright complexion and physical radiance.

Duration of Digestion

The duration for these products to be compiled, i.e. for the nutriment of the food consumed to turn into vital fluid, is six days. However, aphrodisiac compounds, etc. spontaneously develop vital fluid (within one hour of ingestion). Almost all medicines perform their function within one day of ingestion.

HUMORS WHICH INFLICT HARM

The humors which inflict harm have eight aspects: (1) classification, (2) the process of conception, (3) nature, (4) digestive heat, (5) abdomen, (6) location, (7) functions, and (8) characteristics.

Classification

The classification is threefold (according to) wind, bile and phlegm. Their number and order are established on the basis of cause, nature, simile, result and remedy. A body which is stable in its aspects thrives, but if disturbed, it is overcome.

There are five types of wind: (a) life sustaining, (b) ascending, (c) pervading, (d) firelike equalizing and (e) downwards voiding.

The bile classification is also fivefold: (a) digestive, (b) color-transforming, (c) accomplishing, (d) visual, and (e) complex-ion-transforming.

The fivefold classification of phlegm is: (a) supporting, (b) decomposing, (c) experiencing, (d) satisfying, and (e) connecting.

The Process of Conception

The exposition of the process of conception (is as follows): at the first (moment of) conception (the humors) are present in the semen and ovum. For example, this is like an insect developing poison (by evolving from a poisonous tree).

Nature

There are seven natures which (can) come about from humoral excesses due to diet or behavioral pattern when the sperm and ovum are in the womb. If the wind (predominates the child's body will be) small, if bile [predominates his body will be of] medium (size) and if phlegm [predominates his body will be] large. It is best if all three humors (are equally balanced) but (still) fair if any of the three pairs (of humors) are prominent.

Digestive Heat

Thus the digestive heat is fourfold. Because of (the influence of) wind it fluctuates. By (the influence of) bile it becomes sharp and because of phlegm it is weakened. If all three humors (are balanced) it will be even.

Abdomen

(Predominance of) wind makes the stomach firm (internally) and (the influence of) bile loosens the stomach (-motion) (aperient). (If) phlegm (predominates) the stomach will be of medium (tone).

Location

Although the (three humors) abide pervasively throughout the body, in ascending order they abide around the heart and below the navel (wind), between these two (bile), and above (the heart) (phlegm).

Functions of the Humors

The wind performs exhalation and inhalation, articulates (the body), performs actions, firmly expels [mucus, wastes, spittle, etc.] and travels through the objects of harm [e.g., moves blood through veins and arteries], endows the sense organs with clarity, and sustains the body.

The function of the bile is that it gives rise to hunger and thirst, digests food, and provides bodily heat, clear complexion, courage and intelligence.

Phlegm supplies firmness to body and mind, induces sleep, connects the joints (by lubrication), induces patience and lubricates the body, making it smooth.

Specifically the *life-sustaining* wind is located in the crown of the head and travels through the throat and the breastbone, swallows food and drink, inhales, spits, sneezes, belches, endows the mind and sense organs with clarity and holds the mind [and body together].

The *ascending wind* is located in the chest and runs through the nose, tongue and throat. It projects the speech, provides (physical) strength, complexion, 'color,' energy and effort, and clears the memory.

The *pervading wind* is located in the heart and moves throughout the whole body. It raises, presses downwards, moves (the body), stretches, contracts (limbs and digits), opens and closes (the orifices) and is relied upon in the majority of functions.

The *firelike equalizing wind* is located in the stomach and runs throughout the internal (vessel) organs. It digests food, separates nutriment and waste products, and nourishes the objects of harm (bodily constituents, excretions etc.).

The *downwards voiding wind* is located in the anal area and operates in the large intestine, urinary bladder, genitals and thighs. It discharges and retains the semen, (menstrual) blood, stool, urine and fetus.

The *digestive bile* is located between the digested and undigested matter. It digests food, separates the nutriment and waste, produces body heat, assists the remaining four (types of bile) and enhances the strength.

The *color-transforming bile* is located in the liver and transforms all the colors of the nutriment (and other bodily constituents).

The *accomplishing bile* is located in the heart and induces conceptions, pride, intelligence and the fulfillment of desires.

The *visual bile* is located in the eyes and enables one to perceive forms.

The *complexion-clearing bile* is located in the skin and enhances the skin tone.

The *supporting phlegm* is located in the chest, (acts as a) support for the (remaining) phlegms and maintains the moisture (level of the body).

The *decomposing phlegm* abides where (the food is) not (yet) digested. It breaks up and decomposes the food and drink.

The *experiencing phlegm* is situated in the tongue and enables one to apprehend tastes.

The *satisfying phlegm* is located in the head and satisfies the sense organs.

The *connecting phlegm* is located in all the joints, connects the joints and stretches and retracts (the limbs, etc.).

Characteristics

The characteristics of the three humors, wind, bile and phlegm, are (as follows): wind is by nature coarse, light, cold, subtle, firm and mobile; bile is by nature oily, sharp, hot, light, malodorous, aperient and moist; the nature of phlegm is oily, cool, heavy, blunt, smooth, firm and adhesive.

Thus it was said. This concludes the fifth chapter, presenting the physiology of the body, from *The Quintessence Tantra, the Secret Oral Tradition of the Eight Branches of the Science of Healing.*

6. Actions and Classifications of the Body

Then the sage Rig.pahi.ye.she spoke these words: O Great Sage, listen. The actions of the body are physical, verbal and mental, and (consist of) positive, negative and unspecified behavior. In particular the five senses apprehend their respective objects.

There are four classifications of the body (on the basis of gender, age, nature, and disease).

CLASSIFICATION BY GENDER

The threefold classification of gender is male, female and neuter.

CLASSIFICATION BY AGE

The classifications of age are (as follows): Adolescence lasts until the age of sixteen. The bodily constituents, senses, brightness of complexion and physical strength then increase, and adulthood lasts until the age of seventy.[1] From then on in old age the (bodily condition) deteriorates.

CLASSIFICATION BY NATURE

There are seven (types of human) nature including dual and triple combinations (of the humors).

People who are wind-generated are stooped, thin, with dark ('blue') complexion, talkative and unable to endure cold and wind. They shuffle when they walk, have little wealth and short life, are light sleepers and are small in stature. They enjoy laughing, singing, fighting and archery, and prefer sweet, sour, bitter and hot tastes. They possess the characteristics of a vulture, raven and fox.

A bile-natured person has great hunger and thirst, yellow hair and body, sharp mind and great pride. They perspire a great deal, are malodorous, and have medium lifespan, wealth and stature. They prefer sweet, bitter, astringent and cool-powered foods and have the characteristics of a tiger, monkey or 'harmer' spirit.

Phlegm-natured people have cool bodies, joints which are not prominent, corpulence and pale complexion. They have erect posture and can endure protracted hunger, thirst and [the suffering] of mental distortions. They are of stout build, have long lives and much wealth, and are heavy sleepers. (Phlegm people) are not easily roused to anger and are of noble disposition. They prefer hot, sour, astringent and coarse foods and possess the qualities of a lion or 'guardian' buffalo.

[The natures of those influenced by] dual or triple humoral combinations may be understood from combining (the above characteristics).

CLASSIFICATION BY DISEASE

There are undisturbed and disturbed (physical states). The normal state of the body is to remain undisturbed and (thus) one remains free of disease and lives a long life. The body that is afflicted by disease is to be healed.

Thus it was said. This concludes the sixth chapter, presenting the actions and classifications of the body, from *The Quintessence Tantra, the Secret Oral Tradition of the Eight Branches of the Science of Healing*.

7. *Signs of Death*

Then the sage Rig.pahi.ye.she spoke these words: O Great Sage, listen. Omens of death are of four types: distant, imminent, uncertain, and certain.

DISTANT OMENS OF DEATH

The three types of distant omens are of: (1) messenger, (2) dreams, and (3) the malfunctioning (body).

Messenger Omens

A remarkable messenger (e.g., a Tantric practitioner holding a thigh-bone trumpet), a Buddhist monk or corresponding type of person is a sign that the patient will recover. If the opposite is the case [i.e., if the messenger is a woman, neuter, cripple, deformed person or if he rides in on a mule, buffalo, donkey or camel] recovery will not come about.

If the messenger (arrives) frightened, trembling, panting, holding (wood), stone or *bong.wa* (an attractive, roundish but inauspicious stone which varies in color), calling from afar, holding a weapon or stick, wearing a red flower or inauspicious ornaments, or speaking (unfavorably), the task (of healing) will not be accomplished.

It is a sign that the patient will die if the messenger arrives when the doctor has a coarse (irascible) attitude, is speaking (harshly or) inauspiciously, when (grass, etc.) is being cut, when something is being destroyed or when the fire offering of ritual cake for a deceased person is being performed. It is unfavorable if the messenger sets out on the sixth, fourth and ninth days (of the lunar month); during a solar or lunar eclipse; when the stars and planets are unfavorable; or at night. It is an unfavorable sign if whilst (the messenger or the doctor) are on the way something is cut, burned or broken; if either (speaks of or) hears or sees weeping or killing; if a cat, monkey, otter or snake crosses one's path; or if any (other) inauspicious (omen) is seen.

(Auspicious signs:) If while on the way or when about to enter the patient's house, the doctor sees some positive omen—a vessel full of grain, curd etc., a bell, butter lamp, flower, puffed rice, barley flour dough, an image [e.g., a statue of a deity], white ornaments [or clothing], someone engaged in spiritual practice or hoisting a victory banner, something on fire, horses and sheep and cows, etc., with their young, and attractive sounds, food, drink and ornaments—it is a sign that the patient will be cured.

It is an unfavorable sign if curd, the surface film of water on top of curd, (auspicious substances, grains, etc.) are conveyed from the house (of the patient); if a fire (is seen to) die down without (the movement of) the wind; or if a vessel (of any kind) breaks.

Dream Omens

Signs that (the patient) has been seized by the Lord of Death are dreaming that one is riding a cat, monkey, tiger, fox or corpse. (Similarly) one will die if one dreams that one is naked (whilst) riding south on a buffalo, horse, pig, donkey or camel. Signs that one has come under the power of the Lord of Death are (dreaming of): a *lchug.ma* tree[1] (or other type of tree) with a bird's nest in it growing from the crown of one's head; a palmyra tree or other thorny tree growing from one's heart; lotuses emerging (from one's heart); falling over a cliff; sleeping in a cemetery; one's head breaking; being surrounded by crows, hungry ghosts or butchers; the skin falling from one's legs (or arms); entering the mother's womb; being carried away by a river; sinking into a swamp; being swallowed by fish;

receiving iron, gold (or silver); losing in business or battle; at a social gathering being charged an admission fee by dancers (or stage performers); getting married; being naked; having one's hair and beard shaved off; drinking alcohol with deceased relatives or being dragged downwards by them; wearing red clothing or flower garlands and dancing with the dead. Such dreams as these are unfortunate, and a patient will die if he has these dreams continually, due to disease blocking the entrance of the pathway of the consciousness. A healthy person is not certain (to die), for he can be freed (from the influence of such signs) by making religious offerings.

The six types (of dreams) are of: (i) seeing (something perceived during the day), (ii) hearing (any sound heard while awake), (iii) experiencing (a past pleasure), (iv) praying, (v) [dreams containing a corresponding sign that are subsequently] fulfilled, and (vi) (dreams) arising from illness [e.g., blockage of the digestive tract]. No negative effects ensue from all dreams in the first part of the night, nor from dreams which are forgotten. If a dream is seen (upon awakening just after) dawn (and if the mind is) clear, it will bear fruit.

(Fortunate dreams:) whoever dreams of a celestial being (Indra, Brahma, etc.); the leader (-buffalo) of a herd; (holy) or famous men; a blazing fire; a (clear) lake; one's body being smeared with blood or filth; wearing (spotless) white (or yellow) clothing; a banner or umbrella (being raised); receiving fruit; climbing a mountain or (to the top of) a fine house or fruit-laden tree; riding a lion, elephant, horse or ox; crossing a great river or ocean; going towards the north or east; gaining freedom from a miserable (dark place, prison, etc.); defeating an enemy; or of receiving (praise and) veneration from celestials and parents, will gain long life, wealth and freedom from disease.

The Malfunctioning Body

The exposition of death omens according to changes in the character of an ordinary person (is as follows): (If for no reason) one hates one's doctor, medicine, spiritual master, friends and relatives (in spite of cherishing them previously, or vice versa), or if for no reason one becomes conscientious, attractive, healthy or affluent (when previously not so) or vice versa, it is a sign of (imminent) death.

Always (having poor) complexion (like one afflicted by a severe illness); negative, unhappy frame of mind; the crows not eating ritual cakes one has put out for them; water quickly drying or not staying on one's chest after bathing; (one's knuckles) not cracking when one pulls one's fingers; becoming weak in spite of eating well; a change in the odor of the body; and (increased) accumulation or disappearance of lice eggs, are (also signs of) death.

One is said to have fallen prey to the Lord of Death if (the proportion of) one's desire, ignorance and anger becomes the opposite of their previous (level) (i.e., becomes far greater or far less), or if the previous faults in one's behaviour transform into virtues or vice versa.

(Finally) one will die if, when the sun is shining, (one has no shadow); if one's reflection (is not visible in clear) water or in a mirror; or (if in these and) in a clear sky one (sees) one's reflection without head or limbs.

IMMINENT SIGNS OF DEATH

Imminent signs of death are of two types: imminent and extremely imminent.

Imminent Signs of Death

Imminent signs of death include loss of blood from the nine orifices without their having been affected by poison or weapons; immediately forgetting what has been said; retraction of the penis with the scrotum left hanging down or vice versa; the onset of an unusual sound when clearing the throat or when sneezing; not noticing the smell of a butter lamp that has just gone out; lack of sensation if some hair is pulled out; the appearance of a greasy patch on the crown of the head (without oil having been applied externally); an unusual new parting appearing in one's hair or eyebrows; the appearance of a coarse whorl or of lines in the shape of a new moon on the forehead or groin; the five general (types of) object of the sense faculties taking on a false aspect without cause; the appearance of something (previously) non-existent as existent, and vice versa; not being able to see one's wrist when it is pressed between one's eyes; no (appearance of) light when one presses one's eyes; having a fixed stare like a rabbit; (the eyes) becoming retracted in their sockets; or a lack of lustre in the irises.

One will die if one's ears stick to the sides of one's head, if the faint roaring sound is absent (when one covers one's ears) and if vapor rising from one's head casts no shadow.

Additional signs of death are flaring of the nostrils and the formation of pale dried mucous (below them); the middle of the tongue turning dark; the tongue becoming dry and short; inability to speak; the lower lip hanging down and the upper lip being turned up; dust appearing (instantaneously) on one's face; coldness of the breath; the teeth (repeatedly) turning (black with) dirt; breathing out in short gasps (and being unable to inhale); and loss of (body) heat.

Other signs of death are said to be the onset of a fever (internally) whilst the body feels cold (on the outside); shunning heat when suffering from a cold disorder, or similarly shunning cool things when suffering from a fever; the disorder not responding when the (standard) treatment has been given, and the condition responding favorably to the wrong treatment.

EXTREMELY IMMINENT SIGNS OF DEATH

The extremely imminent (signs of death) are the gradual dissolution of the five elements and the five sense faculties. (Firstly), owing to the dissolution of the power of the earth element into the water element, form is no longer perceived (clearly). Through the dissolution of the power of the water element into the fire element, the nine orifices become dry and through the dissolution of the power of the fire element into the wind element, the (body) heat diminishes. Then, because of the dissolution of the wind element into the space element, the respiration ceases.

By virtue of the deterioration of the eye sense base, form is not clearly (apprehendable) and dissolves into sound whilst through the deterioration of the audial sense base, sound is not clearly (heard) and dissolves into smell. Owing to the deterioration of the olfactory sense base, smell is not clearly (apprehended) and dissolves into taste whereas through the deterioration of the gustatory sense base, tastes are not clearly experienced and dissolve into contact. (Finally) because of the deterioration of the tactile sense base, (objects of) touch cannot be felt. [Next when all have dissolved into the life wind and the consciousness, the consciousness leaves the body to take rebirth.]

UNCERTAIN OMENS OF DEATH

Although omens of death appear according to the manifold forms of disease, by dispelling the disease the signs of death will also be dispelled.

CERTAIN OMENS OF DEATH

If the omens remain firm, although (the disease) has been, dispelled then death is certain.

If one's outer, inner and vital constituents, (namely) flesh, nutriment and channels, go into decline and are impaired one is certain to die. Although various methods of treating the disorder (may be applied) to effect a cure, they will be ineffective and death is certain.

When the bodily aggregates are overcome by the omens of death the humors, bodily constituents and excretions are disrupted. This resembles (the way in which) Mount Meru and the rest of the universe are destroyed when the elements undergo transformation. Ignorance of the omens of death prevents (the doctor from knowing when to) agree to or to decline to treat (a patient) and without such knowledge he will not acquire a good reputation. Therefore one who wishes (to be known as) an expert (physician) should know the signs of death.

(The above) omens may be reversed in the case of dreams, character, distant and uncertain signs by accumulating merits (through generosity, etc.), by reading (scriptures), by meditational practices and (by performing the practices of meditational deities, i.e., by tripling one's daily practice of all of these). With respect to imminent and certain signs, one should save from death (animals, etc. that are due to be killed, e.g., by paying for their release). There are (however) no means of reversing extremely close omens.

Thus it was said. This concludes the seventh chapter, presenting the signs of death, from *The Quintessence Tantra, the Secret Oral Tradition of the Eight Branches of the Science of Healing*.

8. *The Causes of Disease*

Then the sage Yid.las.skyes asked, O Master, Sage Rig.pahi.ye.she, how may one learn the principles of the rise and decline of disease? May the Healer, King of Physicians please explain?

At this the Master said, O Great Sage, listen. The instruction in the rise and decline of disease arising from the aggregates (of the body) to be healed is said to be sevenfold, namely,

(1)   causes (chapter eight),
(2)   immediate causes (chapter nine),
(3)   means of entry (of disease) and
(4)   location (chapter ten),
(5)   nature and characteristics (chapter eleven)
(6)   classifications and
(7)   individual significances (chapter twelve).

Causes are twofold: distant and near.

DISTANT CAUSES

Distant causes (in turn) are general and specific. The body has been infinitely afflicted in various ways by humoral imbalances. Since it is not possible (here) to show every single cause, the *general causes* of all disease will be expounded. The sole cause of all disease is said to be ignorance due to lack of understanding of the meaning of selflessness. For example, even a bird soaring in the sky is not separated from its shadow. Even though beings may live and act with contentment, because of possessing ignorance they cannot be separated from disease.

Specific causes: from ignorance arise the three poisons of attachment, hatred and closed-mindedness whence are produced in turn the humors wind, bile and phlegm.

PROXIMATE CAUSES

Undisturbed wind, bile and phlegm are the causes of disease whilst disturbed, imbalanced humors are the nature of disease. They harm the body and life, and give rise to suffering.

Disturbance of the bile burns the bodily constituents. Because it is hot and in the nature of fire, although it abides in the lower body it flares up to the upper (body). All fevers (heat disorders) without exception are produced from it.

A phlegm imbalance smothers the body heat, and being of the nature of earth and water is heavy and cool. Although it is located in the upper body it falls to the lower and all cold disorders arise from it.

Wind pervades both hot and cold: when combined with the sun it assists burning and when in combination with the moon it facilitates cooling. Its movement pervades the whole upper, lower, inner and outer body and imbalances and precipitates both hot and cold disorders. Wind is therefore the cause of all diseases.

Thus it was said. This was the eighth chapter, presenting the causes of disease, from *The Quintessence Tantra, the Secret Oral Tradition Tantra of the Eight Branches of the Science of Healing*.

9. *Immediate Causes of Disease*

Then Sage Rig.pahi.ye.she spoke these words: O Great Sage, listen. There are three conditions which are active in developing the causes (of disease). (These are:) (a) formation increasing conditions, (b) cumulative arising, and (c) (actual) manifesting conditions. Because (the first type) forms and increases (disease) it is called 'formation increasing.' (Because) the second accumulates and (causes disease) to arise, it is called 'cumulative arising.' The third type is (actual) 'manifesting' conditions, so called because they cause the accumulated conditions to manifest.

FORMATION INCREASING CONDITIONS

The formation increasing conditions are season, sensory (experience) and behavioral pattern. Sicknesses are produced if these are inadequate, excessive or perverse.

The three seasons are of heat, cold and rain. They are inadequate if there is little heat, cold or rain and are excessive if there is too much (of any of these in its respective season). They are perverse if there is no [such feature (heat, etc.) in its respective season].

Inadequate (sensory experience) entails little or no contact between the five senses and their objects, whilst extreme application of such means excessive contact. Perverse (sensory) contact is said to be with extremely close, distant, large, small, frightening or unattractive (objects).

Behavior is threefold: physical, verbal and mental. Engaging in little or no activity is inadequate. Engaging in (overly) strenuous activity is excessive, whilst forcefully restraining (some) bodily functions or forcing (others) (e.g., defecation when constipated), twisting (the limbs or body) and other negative actions are perverse.

CUMULATIVE ARISING CONDITIONS

Accumulation, arisal and pacification (of humoral imbalances) are (influenced by) (1) cause, (2) nature and (3) season.

Causes

Causes such as coarse [light, etc.] qualities combined with warmth accumulate a wind disorder, which arises because of cold (conditions) and is pacified by oily, warm (treatment). Similarly a bile disorder is accumulated by sharp [oily, light, malodorous, etc. conditions] combined with coolness, arises because of heat and is pacified by (treatment having) blunt (characteristics) combined with coolness. Heavy and oily [adhesive, blunt, smooth, static, etc. qualities] combined with coolness accumulate a phlegm disorder, which arises through warmth and is pacified by coarse [light, sharp, mobile power].

Nature

(Each humor) increases (in stages) and thus accumulates at its respective location. Humoral disturbances from the above causes (make one) desire (foods, etc.) having the opposite qualities. Upon arisal (the disorder) enters the wrong pathways (locations of other humors) and manifests its own symptoms. It is pacified at its own location to maintain (the right) balance (of humors) and (to ensure) freedom from disease.

Season

The three periods of early summer, [monsoon and autumn] are the times of wind disorders. The bile (season) is late monsoon, [autumn and early winter], (whereas) the season of phlegm disorders is late winter, [spring and early summer].

In early summer wind disorders are accumulated by environmental and bodily factors, diet and behavioral pattern of exclusively light and coarse (nature), but do not arise due to warmth. In monsoon they arise through (the force of) rain, wind and cold and are pacified in autumn by oily, warm (factors).

Bile disorders are accumulated in (late) monsoon by oily factors but cannot arise (because of the) cool conditions. They arise through the oiliness and warmth of autumn and are pacified by the coolness of early winter.

Phlegm disorders are accumulated in late winter by cool oily and heavy factors, but do not arise because they are hidden (by the cold). They arise through the warmth of the spring sun and are pacified by the light, coarse conditions of early summer.

MANIFESTING CONDITIONS

However, although the season of their arisal has not arrived disorders may be precipitated by (factors of) diet and behavioral pattern. Specifically there are two types of immediate conditions: general and specific.

The general conditions which precipitate disease are the season of arisal, spirits, poison, unwholesome food, wrong treatment and the maturation of negative actions.

Specific conditions which give rise to *wind disorders* are excess intake of bitter, light and coarse (foods, etc.), exhaustion from sexual indulgence, lack of food or sleep, extreme exertion of body or speech on an empty stomach, severe loss of blood, being severely affected by diarrhoea and vomiting, being in cool breezes, exhaustion (weeping), grief, intense mental or verbal activity, consumption of non-nutritious food, forcing or forcefully restraining or contracting (mental and bodily functions such as defecating, urinating, sneezing, etc.).

Conditions which cause the heat of *bile disorders* to arise are excess intake of hot-tasting, sharp, hot-powered, oily (foods, etc.); the arisal in the mind of extreme anger; strenuous or violent activity after sleeping on a hot afternoon; carrying excessive loads; digging in hard ground; fighting; ['bending a stiff bow']; racing; fatigue due to walking about while working;

falling from a horse; falling over a cliff; being trapped in a 'cave-in'; being struck by stones or sticks; or excess indulgence in meat, butter, cane sugar, alcohol, etc.

The conditions which precipitate the cold of *phlegm disorders* are excess intake of bitter, sweet, heavy, cool and oily (foods, etc.), relaxing after eating one's fill, sleeping in the daytime or on damp surfaces, catching a chill from wearing thin clothes after bathing, eating freshly picked raw or stale wheat and peas, goat meat, flesh of she-dzo calf, fat, (marrow), seed oil, butter, rotten food, withered leaves, stale radishes, raw hill garlic and sundry raw foods. Also, uncooked or burnt food, (cold) stale food, fresh goat's milk, curd, whey, cold water, tea, and fresh intake of food before an extremely large previous (intake) of food and drink has been digested.

From combinations of the above conditions dual and triple humoral disorders ensue.

Thus it was said. This concludes the ninth chapter, presenting the immediate causes of disease, from *The Quintessence Tantra, the Secret Oral Tradition of the Eight Branches of the Science of Healing.*

10. The Mode of Entry and Locations of Disease

Then the sage Rig.pahi.ye.she spoke these words: O Great Sage, listen. Once a disease has been produced by its causes and conditions its mode of entry is as follows.

THE MODE OF ENTRY OF DISEASE

The four types of conditions [season, spirits, diet and behavioral pattern] fire the projectiles (of the secondary qualities) at the target (of the three humors). One of the targets is struck and (the humors), etc. should be analyzed because of their inter-relationship. Wind is located in the bones, bile in the blood and perspiration, and phlegm in the remaining (bodily constituents). The mode of their mutual dependence is (as follows). A humoral disturbance affects the bodily constituents and both of these (disturbances) then harm the excretions. Moreover the nutriment of food similar in nature (power) to the cause of the disorder is spread to all the cavities (of the body) by the pervading wind. The nutriment then brings about malfunction of whichever cavities it reaches. Just as rain falls when clouds gather in the sky, so (diseases) are accumulated and increased in their own individual locations by behavioral factors. Once an accumulated disorder meets the (appropriate) conditions it must certainly rise. Once it has entered the six pathways [skin, flesh, channels, bones, vital and vessel organs], unhappiness and disease ensue.

LOCATIONS OF DISEASE

Thus, the locations where disease is based once it has entered the body (are as follows): The seats of wind disorders are the post-digestive locations, hip joints, bones, joints, (all areas of) tactile sensation and the ears, and especially in the post-digestive stage, in the large intestine. Bile disorders are located at the navel, in the stomach, blood, perspiration, nutriment, lymph, eyes, skin, and especially between the digested and undigested material in the stomach. Phlegm disorders are situated in the chest, throat, lungs, head, nutriment, flesh, fat, marrow, semen, stool, urine, nose, tongue and especially the upper stomach.

Thus it was said. This concludes the tenth chapter, on the mode of entry of diseases, from *The Quintessence Tantra, the Secret Oral Tradition of the Eight Branches of the Science of Healing.*

11. The Symptoms of Disease

Then the sage Rig.pahi.ye.she spoke these words: O Great Sage, listen. The three essential features of humoral disorders are (a) increase, (b) decrease, and (c) disturbance. The causes and symptoms of increase or decrease of the humors, bodily constituents and excretions will (first) be explained.

Firstly the causes of increase and decrease of the humors are that [the patient finds certain beneficial] food undesirable and [considers certain beneficial] behavior to be unwholesome. (He therefore) avoids these and (the humors) increase. Having demanded (certain wrong) food (which he considers desirable) and (considering certain other wrong) behavior to be beneficial, (the patient) is allowed (such or indulges in such on his own initiative, and the humor(s) having qualities opposite to such food and behavior) are decreased.

Secondly the body heat (in the form of the digestive bile) resides in its own location (between the digested and undigested food) but a portion of it resides in each of the bodily constituents. Its subsiding and flaring bring about increase and decrease (of the bodily constituents. Increase and decrease of) the first (bodily constituent) causes each subsequent one to develop or diminish (correspondingly). Know that [because of such increase and decrease of the humors and bodily constituents] the excretions are suppressed or greatly developed.

SYMPTOMS OF INCREASE

Symptoms of a wind increase are thinness, dark complexion, fondness of warmth, shivering, abdominal distention, constipation, loquacity, vertigo, loss of strength and of sleep, and impairment of the sense organs.

(Signs of) a bile increase are yellowing of the stool, urine, skin and eyes, hunger, thirst, a (rise in) body heat, insomnia and loose motions.

Increase of phlegm results in loss of (body) heat, indigestion, heaviness of the body, pale complexion, lassitude, slackness of the limbs, abundant saliva and mucus, much drowsiness and breathing discomfort. [The symptoms of] an increase in nutriment are similar to those of phlegm.

Increase of blood causes erysipelas, internal abscesses, spleen disorders, leprosy, tumors, disorders of blood and bile jaundice (lit. 'yellow eye'), (swelling and other) ailments of the gums, difficulty in moving (the body) and reddening of the eyes, urine and skin.

(Signs of) increase of flesh are goiter, (glandular) excrescences and enhanced growth of flesh, whilst increase of fat results in fatigue and an abundance of fat on the breasts and belly. Increase of bone entails the growth of surplus bones and teeth, whereas (the symptoms of) increase of marrow are heaviness of the body, weak eyesight and thickness of the joints. Increase in semen produces seminal calculi and attraction to women, whilst increase of stool results in heaviness of the body, abdominal distention and intestinal malfunction. Increase of urine causes urogenital pain and the feeling that one has not urinated (when one has just done so), whereas increase of perspiration (is marked by) profuse sweating, unpleasant body odor and skin disorders. Increase of minor [secretions, e.g., 'sleep', mucus, saliva, ear wax, etc.] gives rise to heaviness, itching and necrosis.

SYMPTOMS OF DECREASE

(The symptoms of) decrease of wind are lack of energy, little (inclination to) speak, physical discomfort, unclear memory and the arisal of symptoms of a phlegm increase.

Decrease of bile causes loss of (body) heat and skin tone, coldness and dark complexion.

Decrease of phlegm is marked by emptiness of its natural seats, dizziness, palpitation and loosening of the joints.

Decrease of nutriment results in emaciation, difficulty in swallowing food, coarseness of the skin and inability to tolerate loud noises. Decrease of blood results in slackness (i.e., emptiness) of the blood vessels, coarseness of the skin and [attraction to] cool [sensation] and sour (foods). Decrease of flesh leads to pain in the limb-joints and the skin adhering to the bones, whilst decrease of fat gives rise to insomnia, emaciation and bluish-grey (skin tone). Decrease of bone causes the hair, teeth and nails to fall out, whereas decrease of marrow is indicated by hollowness (of the bones), vertigo and the formation of cataracts, etc. Decrease of vital fluid produces bleeding (from the genitals) and a burning sensation.

Decrease of stool is marked by rumbling and 'contraction' in the small intestine, (and sometimes the wind) rises resulting in pain in the ribs and heart. Decrease in urine gives rise to discoloration (of urine), dysuria and minimal urination, whilst decrease of perspiration results in cracking of the skin and the hairs on the body stand up and fall out. Know that a decrease of the minor (excretions, such as gall bile, 'sleep' in the eyes, etc.) renders their natural locations empty and light.

Since the bodily constituents depend upon their (respective) excretions, increase of the latter produces (disease) and decrease thereof adversely affects the strength (of the bodily constituents). The essential nutriment [upon which one's life force is based] is reduced by mental suffering (resulting in) fear, emaciation, debility, unhappiness and pale complexion. The (appropriate) medicines to remedy this are milk and soup of [fresh, lean] meat.

SYMPTOMS OF DISTURBANCE

Wind

In a disturbance of the wind humor the pulse is empty and floating whilst the urine is (clear) like water and becomes thin after discoloration. (Other symptoms are) restlessness, protracted sighing, light capricious mind (as reflected in the speech), dizziness like that experienced when intoxicated, humming or buzzing sounds in the ears, dry, red, coarse tongue, astringent taste in the mouth, shifting pains, coldness, shivering, pain throughout the body [when one moves], lethargy, stiffness and shrinking (of limbs), feeling of separation (of flesh from skin and bones) or (as if one's bones) are broken, bulging [sensation in the eyes, etc.], feeling (as if the body has been) bound, great pain when one moves, the raising of the hairs on one's body, formation of goose pimples, insomnia, yawning, trembling, a wish to stretch, short temper, feeling as if the hips, waist, bones and all joints have been beaten, shooting pains below the occiput (in the nape of the neck), in the chest and cheek bones, opening of the secret wind points [sixth and seventh vertebrae] and pain when they are pressed, dry heaves, coughing up soft bubbles around dawn, rumbling of the stomach, and post-digestive pain in the evening and around dawn.

Bile

The symptoms of a bile disturbance are a strong, thin (and taut), rapid pulse; reddish-yellow, malodorous urine with much steam; headaches; heat in the flesh; bitter and sour tastes in the mouth; thick phlegm on the tongue; dry nostrils; and the whites of the eyes (taking on) an orange (hue). Also, shooting pains, insomnia (or little sleep at night) and inability to control (i.e., to prevent) sleep in the daytime, salty, orange mucus (from the throat), great thirst, loose motions and vomiting of bile and blood, profuse sweating, body odor, ripening of orange complexion, necrosing of the body, or pain at noon, midnight and during digestion.

Phlegm

A phlegm disturbance is symptomized by a sunken, weak, slow pulse; pale urine with little odor or steam; inability to taste; pale tongue, gums (and palate); pale swollen eyes; abundant mucus (in nose and throat); 'fogginess' in the head; mental and physical heaviness; anorexia; lack of digestive heat; poor digestive power; pain in the kidneys and waist; distention; goiter; vomiting and loose motions (of food) with phlegm; unclear memory; much sleepiness; lethargy; skin irritation; stiffness; tightness in the joints; weight increase; and procrastination. (Phlegm disorders) arise in wet weather, around dusk, in the morning and immediately after eating.

The above symptoms of increase, decrease and disturbance apply to all diseases. All dual, triple and mixed combinations (of disorders) may be understood from these symptoms and there cannot be any symptoms of disease not included here.

Thus it was said. This concludes the eleventh chapter, presenting the symptoms of disease, from *The Quintessence Tantra, the Secret Oral Tradition of the Eight Branches of the Science of Healing.*

12. The Classification and Individual Significance of Diseases

CLASSIFICATION OF DISEASES

Then the sage Rig.pahi.ye.she spoke these words: O Great Sage, listen. The threefold classification of disease is according to the divisions of (1) causes, (2) the basis (i.e., the patient) and (3) the features (of the disease).

(1) CLASSIFICATION ACCORDING TO CAUSES
   The classification according to causes is threefold: (diseases) arising from: (a) the humors of this life, (b) past (negative) actions, and (c) a combination of both of these.
   The first of these arises through the concurrence of causes and conditions.
   Secondly [disorders] arising from past [negative] actions greatly intensify without (any apparent) cause (and are to be remedied by religious practices as well as by medicines).
   [Disorders arising from] a combination of the humors (of this life and past actions) are greatly intensified by the slightest causes [and conditions].
   [Disorders arising from] the humors of this life are twofold: (i) internal humoral (disorders) inherent to the body, i.e., [from disturbance of] wind, bile and phlegm; and (ii) sudden humoral disorders arising from external conditions, i.e., from poisons, weapons and spirits.

(2) CLASSIFICATION ACCORDING TO THE PATIENT
With regard to the categories of patient, there are the four (specific) types, (a) men, (b) women, (c) children and (d) old people, and a fifth category, general (disorders) common to all.

Men. Disorders in men are said to include both deficiency and excess of semen, swelling of the testicles (according to any of) the six [causal factors of wind, bile, phlegm, fat, urine and small intestine] and nine (disorders) of the penis (making a total of) seventeen.

Women. Gynecological disorders include five womb disorders (caused by wind, bile, phlegm, blood and any combination of these); nine (types of) womb tumor; two types of womb parasites, i.e., ascending and irritation types; and sixteen (types of) channel disorder [related to the lungs, heart, liver, spleen, gall bladder, kidneys, small intestine, (milk), breasts, etc., (and head, bones, heart, kidneys, stomach and large intestine) making a total of] thirty-two.

Children. Children's disorders consist of eight subtle ailments [cranial swelling; quinsy; disorders of the spleen, gall bladder, stomach, and large intestine; dietary imbalance and a breast milk disorder], eight gross ailments [of the chest, lungs, and liver; diarrhoea, vomiting, contagious fevers, disorders of the navel and the formation of calculi] and eight very subtle disorders [of the eyes, ears, nose and mouth, lymph-caused glandular swellings, life-channel disorders, parasites, boils and flesh disorders].

Old people. Diseases in the aged entail the decline in strength of this body [comprising the five] elements.

General disorders. General disorders common to all are classified according to:
    (A) [one hundred and one disorders of] the humors
    (B) [one hundred and one] principal disorders
    (C) [one hundred and one disorders according to] location
    (D) [one hundred and one disorders according to] type.

A.   *Disorders of the Humors*
(Disorders of) the three humors are classified according to
wind, bile and phlegm.
  Wind disorders are twofold: *(a)* general and *(b)* specific.
  (a)   General wind disorders are classified according to both
        type and location:
        (i)   There are twenty wind disorders classified ac-
               cording to type, and
        (ii)   When classified according to location there are
               six types of entrance (of wind disorders) and
               seven with the blooming of the flower (of wind
               disorders) in the five sense organs.
  (b)   There are five specific wind disorders affecting the life-
        sustaining and other (winds) and a further ten are
        presented in combination with phlegm and bile.
Thus there are forty-two categories of wind disorders.
  Bile disorders are twofold: *(a)* general and *(b)* specific.
  (a)   General bile disorders are classified according to both
        type and location:
        (i)   The threefold classification according to type
               consisting of excessive accumulation of bile,
               displacement of bile, and overflow of bile which
               runs into the channels.
        (ii)   The classification according to location is seven-
               fold including the six entrances and the sense
               organs.
  (b)   There are five specific bile disorders affecting the
        digestive and other biles, and a further ten are presented
        in combination with wind and phlegm.
Thus there are twenty-six categories of bile disorders.
  Phlegm disorders are twofold: *(a)* single and *(b)* complex.
  (a)   Single phlegm disorders are of general and specific
        types:
        (i)   General phlegm disorders are classified accord-
               ing to both type and location:
               (a') The six categories according to type com-
                     prise xiphoid process (*lhen,* a disorder in
                     the area of the cardiac sphincter), etc.
               (b') Classification according to location is sev-
                     enfold including the six entrances and the
                     sense organs.

(ii)   There are five specific phlegm disorders affecting the supporting phlegm, etc. and a further ten presented in combination with wind and bile.

(b)   With respect to complex phlegm disorders there are both yellow and brown types, the latter of which is fourfold: *(i)*spreading, *(ii)*increasing, *(iii)*leaking, and *(iv)* inflated.

Thus there are thirty-three categories of phlegm disorders, making a total of one hundred and one disorders of the (three) humors.

B. *Principal Disorders*

Principal disorders are classified according to single and complex.

A single disorder manifests symptoms of (an imbalance of) one individual humor. This entails increase, great increase, extreme increase, decrease, [great decrease and extreme decrease of each humor, making a total of eighteen].

Complex disorders are threefold, namely bi-humoral imbalances, tri-humoral disorders and additional disorders.

(a)   *Bi-humoral disorders* entail the three equal (increases or decreases of two humors at once as well as] the six (instances of) strong [increase or decrease of] one [humor accompanied by] extreme [corresponding increase or decrease] of a second humor. [Examples of the latter would be a strong increase of wind accompanied by an extreme increase of bile, or a strong decrease of wind with an extreme decrease of bile].

(b)   In *tri-humoral disorders* [the three humors are subject to an] equal [collective increase or decrease] plus six combinations of a strong [increase or decrease in] one humor with a medium [increase or decrease of a second humor and a minor increase or decrease of] the third.

[There are also a total of] six [combinations in which there is increase of] two [humors accompanied by an] extreme [increase of] one [humor, and in which there is increase of one humor accompanied by extreme increase of the other two humors]. The reverse [also applies, in terms of] decrease [i.e., decrease of one humor accompanied by extreme decrease of the other two, and decrease of any two humors with extreme decrease of the third].

In the six combinations of associated increase and decrease [the first humor is] balanced, [the second] increases [and the third] decreases.

(Finally) there are six [combinations in which one humor] decreases whilst two increase and in reverse [two humors decrease whilst one increases].

Thus there are seventy-four categories of increase and decrease (of the humors).

(c)   There are three categories of *additional disorders* involving the arisal of any disorder on top of another. These are described as:

   (i)   Entry of any disordered humor(s) into the location of another.

   (ii)   Disturbances of other humor(s) before the disorder of the first one has been pacified.

   (iii)   A reaction between two types of humoral disorders, (e.g., wind retains its natural location and reacts with bile and phlegm, or wind occupies the natural location of bile and reacts with phlegm, etc.)

(Thus (i), (ii) and (iii) comprise) three sets of nine, making a total of one hundred and one principal disorders.

C.   *Disorders Classed according to Location*

With regard to location there are the divisions of body and mind.

(a)   *Disorders located in the mind* are twofold: insanity and amnesia.

(b)   *Disorders located in the body* are fourfold in the upper, lower, outer and inner (parts of the body) with a fifth type, (namely), disorders common to the outer and inner body.

   (i)   (Disorders of) the *upper body* are located in the head and sense organs (and specifically) in the head, eyes, ears, nose, lips, teeth, tongue, palate and goiter.

   (Disorders) located in the throat and above the neck are fourfold including [general throat] disorders (e.g., tonsillitis), blockage [e.g., due to tumors in the throat], constriction of the throat [e.g., due to quinsy, diphtheria, etc.] and hoarseness.

Disorders located generally above the neck are fivefold: [extreme] thirst, hiccoughs, asthma, anorexia and the common cold, making a general total of eighteen types.

(ii) The presentation of *internal disorders* affecting the vital and vessel organs is elevenfold: i.e. disorders of the heart, lungs, liver, spleen, kidneys and of the stomach, gall bladder, small and large intestines, urinary bladder and seminal vesicle.

Disorders generally located in the vital and vessel organs are sixfold: indigestion, abdominal cramps, tumors, *sur.ya* (tumorous abscesses), cholera and colic. Disorders generally located in the vessel organs are twofold—diarrhoea and vomiting—thus making a total of nineteen types of disorder.

(iii) Disorders of the *lower body* are fivefold: hemorrhoids, anal fistula, constipation, urinary blockage and diuresis.

(iv) Disorders located in the *outer body* (are found in) the skin, flesh, channels and bones.

(a') Ten skin diseases are set forth: *(sha.bkra)* leucoderma, (in which the skin discolors in patches); *bas.ldags* (with pale complexion and pimples); *gyan.pa* (itching, cff. scabies); *glang.shu* (similar to *bas.ldags* with small sores); *za.kong* (a highly contagious condition involving loss of hair from the pores and bluish complexion); *shu.wa* (in which the skin is coarse and cracked with either a hot sensation or a cold, itching sensation), cff. eczema, venereal diseases, warts; *ngo.khab* (with dark patches on the face), and other disorders which spread in the skin.

(b') Flesh disorders are threefold: goiter, *rmen.bu* (lumps appearing in the glands because of disordered lymph) and other disorders which develop in the flesh.

(c') Disorders of the channels are threefold: *rtsa.dkar* (including polio, Parkinson's disease and other forms of paralysis); *rtsa.nag* (lit., 'black channel') and other disorders which circulate in the channels. Rheumatism is located throughout the bones, flesh, (channels and skin). These come to an overall total of twenty.

(d') Bone disorders are also threefold, including both gout, *rkang.bam* (includes elephantiasis), and other disorders which adhere to the bones.

(v) Disorders which pervade the *outer and inner* (parts of the body) include bile disorders; 'brown [phlegm]'; first, second and third stages of oedema; consumption; the six categories of fever [unripened fever, high fever, empty fever, hidden fever, chronic fever and 'turbid' fever]; spreading fever; disturbed fever; contagious fever; poxes; *'lhog.pa'* (e.g., diphtheria); poisoning by compounded poisons; from toxins (carried in) the air; from (the sun's) rays; vapor poisoning; meat poisoning; poisoning from unwholesome (food combinations); Aconite poisoning; rabies poisoning; poisoning from insects and from snakebites; disorders caused by bhuta *(hbyung.po)* spirits; by planetary influences; leprosy; sores which ulcerate; erysipelas; parasites; sores on the head; thoracic disorders; disorders of the limbs and neck.

These come to a total of thirty-seven, making a grand total of one hundred and one diseases classified according to location.

D. *Disorders Classed according to Type*

With regard to type there are the four divisions of internal disorders, lesions, fevers and miscellaneous disorders.

(a) The divisions of *internal disorders* are twofold: the causal indigestion and the chronic consumptive disorders resulting therefrom.

(i) *Indigestion* is fourfold: its nature, type, accompanying factors and stage.

(ii) The resultant *chronic consumptive disorders* are classified according to both fresh and advanced types.

(a')' The fresh onset type has four aspects: a single phlegm disorder, brown phlegm, a bile disorder and a chronic consumptive disorder caused by poisoning.

(i') Single phlegm disorders are sixfold: disorders of the xiphoid process, the 'iron dirt' syndrome (referring to discoloration of the abdomen), loss of digestive heat, throat constriction, 'white' rheumatism and *hju.ske.ma* (a malnutrition syndrome due to the presence of parasites related to phlegm).

(ii') Brown phlegm disorders are tenfold: 'spreading', 'developed,' 'punctured,' 'ruptured,' 'inflated' (lit., 'swirling'), 'rolled,' 'hidden,' 'reactive,' 'falling into the vessels' and 'intractable cold'.

(iii') The three (chronic) consumptive bile disorders (induced by indigestion) are (1) overflow of bile, (2) which runs into the channels and (3) displacement of bile.

(iv') Chronic consumptive disorders caused by poisoning [and resulting in indigestion] (arise from) both hot and cold (-powered) compounds.

(b') The five types of advanced chronic (consumptive disorders) comprise tumors, the three stages of oedema, and pulmonary tuberculosis.

(i') The eight types of tumor are said to be

of blood, gall bile, xiphoid process, calculi, wind, parasites, channels and urinary tract.

(*ii'*) Third stage oedema is of four types: spreading, 'dripping,' 'swirled fluid,' and 'puncture-fluid.'

(*iii'*) Second stage of oedema is of both hot and cold types.

(*iv'*) First stage oedema is fivefold: of lungs, heart, liver, spleen and lymph.

(*v'*) Pulmonary tuberculosis is fourfold, i.e., of wind, bile, phlegm and supplementary types.

Thus the overall total of internal disorders is forty-eight.

(*b*) *Lesions* include (eruptions) arising from internal factors and (wounds) of an adventitious nature.

(*i*) (Skin) eruptions include sores, *rmen.bu* (glandular lumps caused by disordered lymph), *sur.ya* (abscesses caused by tumoral growths in the ducts of the organs), erysipelas, hemorrhoids, *rkang.bam* (e.g., elephantiasis) and anal fistula. (Hydrocele may also be counted in this section.)

(*ii*) *Wounds* are classified according to location and type.

(*a'*) The locations are the head, neck, abdomen and limbs.

(*b'*) The eight types of wound (occur through) 'peeling,' splitting, severing, (the injured part being) suspended (after being partially severed), amputation, stabbing, splitting and fracturing (of bones).

These make a sum total of fifteen categories (of lesion).

(*c*) (The different types of) *fever* include (*i*) unripened fever, (*ii*) high fever, (*iii*) 'empty fever,' (*iv*) 'hidden fever,' (*v*) chronic fever, and (*vi*) turbid fever; plus the four types known as (*vii*) 'spreading fever,' (*viii*) 'disturbed fever,' (*ix*) contagious fever, and (*x*) poisoning-fever.

(*vii*) Spreading fever is of both external (in skin and flesh) and internal (in vital organs) types.

(*viii*) Disturbed fever is of high, empty or mild types

(according to the influence of bile, wind and phlegm respectively).

(ix) Contagious fevers are of five types: *bal.nad* (a contagious disorder affected by an imbalance of each of the humors), colic, poxes, *gag.lhog* (includes diphtheria, quinsy, etc.) and the common cold.

(x) Poisoning (-fever) is caused by three factors; compounded poisons, food poisoning and natural poisons.

(d) The nineteen *miscellaneous disorders* are hoarseness, hiccoughs, anorexia, (severe) thirst, asthma, cramps, parasites, diarrhoea, vomiting, constipation, anuria, polyuria (includes diabetes), gastroenteritis, gout, rheumatism, lymph disorders, 'white channel' (includes polio, Parkinson's disease, etc.), skin diseases and minor disorders.

Thus there are one hundred and one diseases classified according to type, and four hundred and four disorders in the four divisions of humors, principal disorders, type and location.

These also include (1) disorders (influenced by other karmic factors) which prove fatal despite treatment, (2) disorders (caused by) spirits imputed (by the mind) and from which one is freed by rituals, (3) disorders brought about [by the humors of this life] which prove fatal if not treated (whereas) with treatment the patient will live, and (4) [disorders having only the appearance of disease from which] one recovers naturally without treatment.

If one applies these four categories to each one (of the four divisions above) there will be four hundred and four (in each division) making a combined total of one thousand six hundred and sixteen.

(3) CLASSIFICATION ACCORDING TO THE FEATURES OF DISEASE

In terms of the different aspects (of disease) there are countless divisions. There are twenty-five humors and objects of harm (bodily constituents and excretions), and since numerous kinds of single, dual and triple humoral disorders occur, no fixed enumeration or names are presented. However, the number of humors to be afflicted is not more than three, and there are no locations of disease other than the ten objects of harm. For example, wherever birds may (wish to) fly there is nowhere for them to fly other than the sky. Similarly, since phlegm and wind are (by nature) cold, and bile and blood are hot, despite the numerous categories (of diseases) they are all contained within the two (divisions of) hot and cold.

INDIVIDUAL SIGNIFICANCES OF DISEASE

In the case of (each) individual (disorder) there are the four (stages of) cause, early stage, the manifest stage and the 'overflow' stage:

The cause is the actual condition which produces disease.

In the so-called early stage the specific (symptoms) are still unclear.

The manifest stage is when the symptoms of the actual disease become clear.

The 'overflow' stage is when the disorder has reached its peak and is at full strength in its own location.

With regard to the enumeration, diagnosis, principal (divisions of) and strength (of disease);

The enumeration contains the divisions of the particular types of disease.

Diagnosed disorders are classified (individually) without being mixed.

The principal [divisions of disease] are single and complex including initial and additional disorders.

The strength (of the disease will be) either (great or small) according to the influence of the environment, season, (humoral) nature (of the patient), age group, (humoral) type of disorder, diet and behavioral pattern.

Thus it was said. This concludes the twelfth chapter, presenting the classification of diseases, from *The Quintessence Tantra, the Secret Oral Tradition of the Eight Branches of the Science of Healing*.

13. Routine Behavior

Then the sage Yid.las.skyes asked: O Master, Sage Rig.pahi.ye.she, how may one learn the principles of (healthy) behavior? May the Healer, King of Physicians please explain.

At this the Master said: O Great Sage, listen. The instruction in the principles of behavioral pattern which act as a remedy for healing disease is threefold:

(1)   Routine behavioral pattern (chapter thirteen),
(2)   Seasonal behavioral pattern (chapter fourteen),
(3)   Incidental behavioral pattern (chapter fifteen).

Of these, the activity of routine daily life [is threefold]: (a) [activity geared to] this life alone, (b) worldly (activities), and (c) sacred activity.

ROUTINE ACTIVITY GEARED TO THIS LIFE

First with respect to behavior geared to this life alone, for those who wish to enjoy continual happiness and long life there are the supreme medicines (precious pills, etc.), gemstones and the wearing of amulets consecrated by secret mantras.

Always be mindful to avoid the two manifesting conditions of disease [i.e., wrong diet and behavioral pattern]. Avoid negative actions of body, speech and mind, and devote yourself to immaculate [behavior]. One should never torment one's sense of taste, etc., nor overindulge (the senses) with pleasures. Avoid (sailing in) suspect boats, riding untamed animals, places where killing [and banditry occur], (entering) vast (stretches of) water or banks of flame, climbing on cliffs in monsoon and to the tops of trees in wintertime. If staying in a place one should examine it, and on going one should check the way. [One should not travel] at night (but if) an important reason [necessitates this then] one should carry a stick and proceed with a companion.

Because not sleeping at night has a coarse effect on the body one should sleep in a comfortable position. If one misses (a night's) sleep one should fast all morning and sleep for half (a normal night's sleep). Because of the coarseness and short nights of early summer the body is deprived of strength, wind is increased and therefore it is beneficial to sleep a little in the daytime.

(It is recommended) to eat oily, heavy foods if one has been intoxicated, is very low on energy, exhausted due to grief or exertion, (after) prolonged speech, in old age, or if one has been very frightened.

Otherwise sleeping in the daytime increases phlegm, induces swellings, dullness (of mind), headaches, lethargy, and susceptibility to infectious fevers. For (persistent) oversleeping one should apply an emetic, fast and enjoy the company of women. For insomnia drink milk, curd, alcohol, meat soup, rub [e.g., sesame oil] on the head and pour a little oil in the ears.

Refrain from intercourse with non-humans, another's spouse, one who is unattractive, a pregnant woman, or someone who is very weak, ill or having a period (as this can cause illness to both man and woman because of the impure blood). In winter when the sperm is generated with vigor there are no restrictions (on intercourse). In autumn and spring (every) two days [is the recommended maximum frequency of intercourse] and during monsoon and early summer (only) every fifteen days (is the recommended frequency). Otherwise more frequent intercourse with women dulls the senses and causes dizziness and ultimately demise.

Regular massage with oil overcomes ageing, fatigue and wind disorders. [Periodic] application (of oil) on the head, feet and ears induces lightness of the body, loss of fat, vitality and increases digestive heat. [Physical] toughness and efficiency result from taking proper exercise.

However, by excess or improper indulgence in [physical exertion, the body] becomes unworkable. Especially the aged, children, and wind and bile patients should avoid such [unbalanced behavior].

Phlegm patients should take exercise, and strong people and those who eat oily food should exercise in the winter and spring. Then (one should) rub an application [of pulse-flour] on the body and then wipe the body so as to remove phlegm, digest fats, provide clear skin and extremely firm limbs.

[Regular] bathing increases virility, body heat, physical strength, life span and complexion, and dispels itching due to perspiration, lethargy, thirst and excess of body heat. Washing the head in warm water causes hair loss and weakens the eyesight. Bathing should be avoided immediately after meals and by those suffering from fever with dysentery, distention of the abdomen, common cold, indigestion, nose or eye disorders.

The eyes being in the nature of the fire element are impaired by the (satisfying) phlegm, and tears flow as a result. Therefore one should administer the eye medicine, concentrate of Barberry bark, externally, regularly once every seven days as a lacrimator.

Against the enemy of the five sudden ailments one should rely on the friends (i.e., supreme medicines, gemstones, amulets, etc.).

One should adhere impartially not only to one but to all of the above indications. Thus, day or night, whether abiding or travelling one should discard suffering through close application of mindfulness.

WORLDLY ACTIVITIES

Living according to the codes of conduct of the world is the foundation of all good qualities. One should firmly keep one's promise in practice, repay [kindness and debts to others] according to one's word. Although one may have promised (to commit) an evil action one should refrain from doing it and noble actions should be brought to completion even if they are obstructed (by others). Before acting one should examine [the situation] and then perform well [whatever is] beneficial.

One should never accept a profusion of statements as true, (but only) accept them after examining them thoroughly. One should (first) express the many things one has to say in one's mind and then summarize one's main points (verbally). Never listen to the talk of women and be close-mouthed on confidential matters, but to those who love one and on whom one depends one should speak freely without using deceitful words. Also be gentle and controlled but spontaneously friendly and happy.

One should not leave openings for one's enemies but bide one's time and subdue them with (skilful) means.

One's relatives and attendants should be cared for with affection and one should long remember the past kindnesses (of others). To one's Teacher, father, [mother], uncles, elders of the family, etc., one should respectfully offer service. Let one's thoughts accord with one's compatriots, friends, relatives and others with whom one must associate.

One should be thrifty [in farming and business in general], but when it is necessary one should [give and spend] liberally. When in the wrong one should readily admit defeat and when successful one should be satisfied. If one is learned one should subdue one's pride and if wealthy be contented. One should not be contemptuous towards subordinates and avoid being envious of superiors. One should never support evil people nor take sorcerers as enemies. Never deprive others of their wealth [for harm done to others rebounds upon oneself] and refrain from uttering curses (about trivial things). (In all situations) one should step cautiously so as to avoid regret (later) and never entrust power to evil people.

One's mind should be powered by honesty and one should develop a foundation of forbearance and broad-mindedness. As a rule one should gladly accept tasks according to the amount of time available.

If such a person (who adheres to this code) is reborn as an only child he will not lose his power to others and even if (he takes) the form of a servant he will become the master of many.

SACRED ACTIVITY

Since all sentient beings desire happiness, they engage in all (kinds of) activities. However if they do not (practice) the

Doctrine, their very (contaminated) happiness will become a cause for suffering. Therefore one should make effort in (the practice of) the Doctrine, devote oneself to one's spiritual master, and give other (negative) people a wide berth.

With body, speech and mind refrain from the ten negative actions of (1) taking life, (2) stealing, (3) sexual misconduct, (4) lying, (5) idle gossip, (6) harsh speech, (7) divisive speech, (8) covetousness, (9) malice, and (10) distorted views.

(Moreover) one should render service in every possible way to those (suffering) misery, disease, poverty and pain. Always regard worms, insects and the like as being similar to oneself (in desiring happiness and in being averse to suffering). Smile gently (at others) without deceit and speak truthfully. One should benefit in particular the enemies who endeavor to do one harm, and with love (for all beings) generate the two [aspiring and engaging] supreme Awakening Minds. Subdue the body, speech and mind, have a generous attitude without any sense of a loss and consider the welfare of others as being like one's own. These are the ideals of religious behavior.

Thus it was said. This concludes the thirteenth chapter, on routine daily behavior, from *The Quintessence Tantra, the Secret Oral Tradition of the Eight Branches of the Science of Healing.*

14. Seasonal Behavior

Then the sage Rig.pahi.ye.she spoke these words: O Great Sage, listen. Secondly, seasonal behavior (is explained according to the six seasons of the year): (1) early winter, (2) late winter, (3) spring, (4) summer, (5) monsoon, and (6) autumn.

(Starting in the) first winter month, each season in turn is of two months' [duration]. [One hundred and twenty mental impulses make] one instant, [sixty of which make] one 'minute.' [Thirty 'minutes' make] one 'hour' [and thirty 'hours' make] one day [twenty-four hours]. [Thirty days make] one month [and two months make] one season, [six of which make] one year.

The sun turns about [daylight begins to increase or decrease] eleven days after the solstices of the preceding year. [But, e.g., if the preceding year's solstice was on the twenty-third of the Tibetan month (or after), the total including eleven extra days would be thirty-four. In this case one takes the second digit as being the date and so the fourth day of the fifth Tibetan month would be the summer solstice. This principle applies if the previous year's solstice was on the twentieth of the month or after.] Therefore it is said that for three seasons the sun moves south and for three to the north. Half way [through each cycle of three seasons, i.e., at the equinoxes] night and day are of equal duration. Eighteen [days after the vernal equinox] the sound [of thunder] booms forth and ceases [eighteen days after the autumn equinox].

Moreover during the last month of winter and thereafter as the sun moves towards the north, the power of the wind [element] and sun will assume a sharp, hot, coarse nature and will consume [the cool, oily] qualities of the moon and earth [element]. At that time the extremely powerful flavors of hot, astringent and bitter daily deprive men of their strength and vigor. During the monsoon [and thereafter, as the sun] travels southward, one's strength again increases as the cool [quality of the earth element and] the power of the moon prevail, and the [sharp, hot, coarse powers of] the sun decline. The heat of the land is pacified by the wind and rainfall, and sour, salty and sweet tastes increase in power. In the winter one's strength is at its peak, at its lowest in summer and monsoon, and medium in spring and autumn. Thus the presentation of the two phases of the sun's course is concluded.

Next, with respect to behavioral pattern during the six seasons: in early winter due to the cold the pores constrict, and as the power of the [internal] heat and the [equalizing] wind is boosted, if one's food intake diminishes the bodily constituents deteriorate. Therefore one should rely on [foods having] the first three tastes [sweet, sour and salty]. At this time since the nights are long one becomes hungry [early in the morning], and because the bodily constituents deteriorate [through the powerful digestive heat having nothing to act upon] one should apply [externally] sesame oil, [or other seed oils] and take meat soup and oily [foods]. One should always wear [warm clothing such as animal] skins and shoes, moderately warm oneself by [hot] fomentation, by a fire or by the sun's rays and live in an earthen house having [walls] of double [thickness]. Since it is exceedingly cold in late winter, following the above behavioral pattern is recommended.

In the (late) winter phlegm accumulates in the abdomen and in the springtime the digestive heat declines because of the rays and warmth of the sun. The phlegm then rises [further impeding digestion] and so one should rely on [foods having] the last three tastes [bitter, hot and astringent]. One should partake of old barley [roasted], meat of dry land animals, honey, [hot] boiled water, and ginger decoction, i.e., rely on coarse [-powered foods and drinks]. Vigorous walking and rubbing [pea-] flour [on the skin] cure phlegm imbalances and one should sit in fragrant, shady groves.

In early summer since the great heat of the sun's rays deprives one of strength one should take sweet, light, oily and cool [-powered] foods. Avoid salty, hot [-tasting], sour foods, exertion and [exposure to] the sun. One should bathe in cool water and only drink alcohol [when it is] mixed with water. Wear very thin clothing and dwell in a cool, fragrant house. [Finally] one should sit in the shade of trees [with glossy leaves], in moist winds and cool, fragrant [southern] breezes.

In the monsoon clouds gather in the sky and [the land is] moistened by the rain. The wind, cold, vapor from the earth, and contaminated water impair the digestive heat, and so one should rely on heat-producing (foods). Eat foods having the first three tastes [sweet, sour and salty] and light, warm and oily powers; drink alcohols made from grain grown in dry areas, avoid cool (places such as) the roof of one's house and remain [in warm surroundings].

In monsoon [the power of the rain and wind] is cool but immediately [afterwards] one's body is scorched by the sun's rays. The bile which has accumulated in the rainy season rises in the autumn and to dispel it one should rely on sweet, bitter and astringent foods. Wear clothing scented with camphor, [white] sandalwood and *khus khus* (grass) and frequent rooms sprinkled (with cooling fragrances and water). In short take warm-powered food and drink during monsoon and winter, coarse (diet) in spring, and cool [food] in early summer and autumn.

In monsoon and winter take (foods having) the first three tastes [sweet, sour and salty] and in spring use the last three tastes [bitter, hot and astringent]. In early summer eat sweet things and in autumn rely on sweet, bitter and astringent diet. Take aperient medicines in autumn and emetics in the spring, whilst suppositories are recommended in monsoon. If [the treatment is] inadequate, excessive or misdirected then one should apply the appropriate treatment [to any new syndrome that arises as a result].

Thus it was said. This concludes the fourteenth chapter, on seasonal behavioral patterns, from *The Quintessence Tantra, the Secret Oral Tradition of the Eight Branches of the Science of Healing.*

15. Incidental Behavioral Patterns

Then the sage Rig.pahi.ye.she spoke these words: O Great Sage, listen. Thirdly the presentation of incidental behavior is as follows: do not obstruct the impetus of hunger, thirst, vomiting, yawning, sneezing, breathing, sleep, mucus, saliva, stool, gas, urine and semen.

Denying oneself food leads to physical deterioration, debility, [anorexia] and vertigo, and [as a remedy] one should introduce light, oily, warm [-powered] foods in small quantities. Denying oneself drink results in dryness of the mouth, vertigo, heart diseases and disorientation; all cooling factors will prove beneficial.

Suppressing vomiting gives rise to anorexia, asthma, first stage oedema, erysipelas, cutaneous itch, abscesses, leprosy, eye diseases, sputum and contagious disorders. (As a remedy) one should fast, inhale the strong smoke [of sandalwood or eaglewood] or rinse out the mouth [with a decoction of such woods].

Suppression of sneezing leads to loss of clarity of the sense organs, headaches, stiffness of the neck, slanting of the mouth and jaw fractures [due to a wind disorder]. These may be cured by inhaling smoke (as above), taking nasal medicines and looking at the sun.

By suppressing yawning results occur [similar to those of suppressing sneezing] and any methods normally applied to treat wind disorders will prove beneficial.

Suppressing panting when tired [e.g., after exertion] results in tumors, heart diseases and disorientation. In such cases one should rest [and any methods for correcting wind increase will be beneficial].

Denying oneself sleep gives rise to much yawning, lassitude, heaviness of the head, cataracts and indigestion. Drinking meat soup and alcohol, (oil-)massage and sleep will prove beneficial.

Failure to clear the throat of sputum will increase its accumulation (and lead to) asthma, emaciation, hiccoughs, heart diseases and congestion of the oesophagus. For this apply the (standard) means of removing sputum, [e.g., by using wild ginger, longpeper and raw cane sugar].

Retention of saliva produces pain in the heart and head, loss of fluid through the nostrils, vertigo and congestion of the oesophagus. In this case drinking alcohol, sleeping and pleasant conversation are beneficial.

[Forcibly] withholding intestinal gas brings about dryness of stool, constipation, inability to expel gas, tumors, (shooting) pains [in the abdomen], weak eyesight, deterioration of body heat and heart diseases.

Suppression of bowel movement causes waste material to be regurgitated, aching in the brain, anterior transposition (of the calf muscle), influenza and the same syndromes as above [resulting from withholding intestinal gas].

(Forcibly) withholding urine gives rise to calculi, disorders of the urinary tract, of the male genitals, the thighs and also the above disorders (arising from intestinal gas suppression). As a remedy for these one should administer suppositories, apply medicinal baths, (embrocation), (oil) massage, fomentation and medicinal oils (taken internally).

Forcefully withholding semen leads to (involuntary) emission, disorders of the male genitals, anuria, increase of calculi and emasculation. Therefore one should apply suppositories, embrocations, gain intimacy with a woman, take sesame oil, milk, chicken and alcohol.

By suppressing these impulses or by forcing them all kinds of disorders [e.g., contagious fevers] arise and the winds are immediately disrupted. Therefore administer (appropriate) foods, drinks and medicines [as remedies] for [a wind disorder].

Although any disorder may be alleviated by fasting or by (other methods of) pacification, traces of the disorder can recur. Only by thorough purgation (or emesis) can recurrence of the disorder be prevented. Therefore cold (phlegm) disorders accumulated in winter should be purged [by emesis when they arise] in the spring. (Wind) disorders accumulated during summer should be dispelled [by suppository when they arise] in monsoon and [bile disorders] accumulated in monsoon should be expelled by purgation in autumn. Thus by thorough purging, etc., even the remnants of disease are eradicated and one becomes free of disease. One who always adheres to healthy diet and behavior and relies upon an experienced physician will not fall ill. Therefore so that no disease will occur or for pacifying any that do develop, the above modes of incidental behavior are recommended.

Thus it was said. This concludes the fifteenth chapter, on incidental behavioral patterns, from *The Quintessence Tantra, the Secret Oral Tradition of the Eight Branches of the Science of Healing.*

16. Principles of Diet: Normal Diet

Then the sage Yid.las.skyes asked: O Great Sage Rig.pahi.ye.she, how may we learn about the principles of a wholesome diet? We request the physician, the Sovereign Healer, to explain.

At this the Teacher replied: O Great Sage, listen. Of the remedial agents for healing disease one should learn the fundamentals of wholesome diet. Healthy food, drink and activity sustain the body and life-force. Inadequate, excessive or inappropriate (wrong) diet, etc., result in disease and promptly deprive one of life. Therefore one should be sure to gain a thorough knowledge of how to combine food and drink (in the right way). Diet may generally be summarized in a threefold way:

(1) Normal diet (chapter sixteen),
(2) Dietary restrictions (chapter seventeen), and
(3) Partaking of the correct amount of food (chapter eighteen).

Normal diet is twofold: (a) foods and (b) beverages.

FOODS

Food is sub-divided into five types: (1) grain, (2) meat, (3) oil, (4) [cooked] vegetables and (5) prepared foods.

Grains

Grains are in two sections: (a) cereals, and (b) legumes (pulses).

Cereals include rice, millet, 'sixty-day' barley, wheat, barley, coarse thick barley, and wild barley. The pre- and post-digestive tastes of these are sweet. These grains increase semen, cure wind disorders, increase phlegm and act as a tonic. Of these rice is greasy, smooth, cool and light (in its power) and eliminates (disorders of) all three humors, increases semen and stops vomiting and diarrhoea. Millet is heavy and cool; it stimulates growth and heals fractures. Sixty-day barley is cool, light and coarse and relieves anorexia. Wheat is heavy, cool and nutritive; it eliminates wind and bile (disorders). Barley is heavy and cool; it increases peristalsis and is an outstanding tonic. Thick-shelled barley and wild barley are cool and light and cure phlegm and bile disorders.

Legumes (pulses) are of two types: round and flat. Both are astringent, sweet, cool, light and absorbent, and they constrict the openings of the channels. They also eliminate phlegm and fever, stop diarrhoea, remove grease and are beneficial in the [excess] formation of blood, bile or fat when used as an embrocation.

Chickpea is effective against a combination of phlegm and wind, and against hemorrhoids and semen stones. It is used as an expectorant and in asthma, and it increases blood and bile. Black chickpea reduces wind and is a tonic which increases phlegm, bile and semen.

Red dal is astringent and sweet and increases all the three humors. A paste of this dal cures erysipelas, gout affecting the toe; and blood disorders.

Sesame seeds have a heavy and warm power that can cure wind disorders and are aphrodisiac.

Linseed is sweet, bitter, oily and smooth and is beneficial in wind disorders.

Buckwheat has a cool and light power that heals wounds and increases the three humors.

Fresh grains have moist and heavy powers, whilst ripened grains are dry, and old grains are light in power. Raw, cooked and prepared grains are in turn lighter and more readily digested.

Meats

Meats are classified into nine sections (including dry land, aquatic and amphibious animals):

(a) Creatures which dig with their claws; for example, peacock, white grouse *(Tetragallus himalayensis)*, *Perdix daurica,* partridge *(Pyrrhocorax pyrrhocorax)*, jackdaw and hill birds.

(b) Creatures which excavate the earth with their beaks; these include parrot, cuckoo *(Cuculus canorus)*, stockdove, magpie, *Pomatorhinus swinhoei* and sparrow.

(c) Game animals include deer *(Cervus elaphus)*, musk deer, *Procapra pictaudata, Ovis ammon,* rabbits and saiga tatarica *(Pantholops hodgsoni)*.

(d) Larger hill and game animals include saiga antelope *(Nemorhaedus cripus),* spotted deer *(Capreolus capreolus L.* or *Muntiacus reevesi),* wild goat, wild boar, buffalo, rhinoceros, bamboo forest tiger *(Neofelis nebulosa),* wild ass *(Equus hemionus),* wild yak (takin) and wild dzo.[1]

(e) Carnivorous animals include the tiger, leopard, bear *(Selenarctos thibetanus),* snow bear *(Ursus arctos),* snow leopard *(Panthera pardus),* wolf, lynx, fox, hill dog and weasel.

(f) Birds of prey include the vulture, red vulture, harrier hawk *(Milvus Korschun lineatus),*[2] crow, owl and sparrowhawk.

(g) Domestic animals include the dzo, yak, camel, horse, donkey, bull, *skom.po* (the calf of a bull and a dzo), goat, sheep, dog, pig, chicken, cat, etc.

(h) Burrowing animals include the marmot *(Marmota bobak),* porcupine, frog, snake, Tibetan badger, lizard *(Eremias argus),* gecko,[3] and scorpion.

(i) Animals which live in wet places include the crane *(Grus siberica),* swan, red wild duck (sheldrake) *(Tadorna ferruginea),* heron *(Larus canus kamtschatschensis* or *Phalacrocorax carbo sinensis),* bittern *(Anas platyrhynchos* or *Mergus merganser),* otter and fish.

All the different types of meats in the above eight sections[4] are sweet tasting and have a sweet post-digestive taste. They are again classified into initial, intermediate and final sections, these being dry land, aquatic and amphibious types. The flesh of dry land animals has cool, light and coarse powers which eliminate wind and phlegm fevers. The flesh of aquatic animals has oily, heavy and warm powers and is beneficial in disorders of the stomach, kidneys and waist, and in cold wind disorders. The flesh of amphibians has both varieties of power, whereas birds of prey utilize their versatility and strength, and live on raw flesh. Their flesh has coarse, light and sharp powers which increase the digestive heat, disperse tumors, increase flesh and eliminate all cold disorders.

Mutton is oily and warm in power, acts as a tonic, develops the bodily constituents, dispels wind and phlegm and sharpens the appetite. Goat meat is heavy and cool, raises the three humors and is beneficial in syphilis, smallpox and burns. Beef is cool and oily and dispels wind fever. The rump meats of horse, wild ass and donkey dry up pus and eliminate disorders of the kidneys and waist, as well as cold disorders and lymphatic ailments.

Pork is cool and light, heals wounds and eliminates brown phlegm. Buffalo meat is a soporific and increases flesh. Yak meat is greasy and warm, eliminates cold disorders and increases blood and bile.

Flesh of chicken and sparrow increases semen and is beneficial for wounds. Peacock flesh is beneficial in eye diseases, hoarseness and for rejuvenation.

Wild yak meat eliminates cold disorders of the stomach and liver and boosts the digestive heat. The meat of hill and game animals is cool and light, and eradicates fever accompanied by wind or phlegm. Rabbit meat is coarse, increases digestive heat and stops diarrhoea. Marmot meat is greasy, heavy and warm and is beneficial in abscesses; it eradicates cold wind and disorders of the stomach, kidneys, waist and head.

Otter flesh is an aphrodisiac and dispels cold of the kidneys and waist. Fish eliminates stomach disorders, improves the appetite, enhances the clarity of the vision and heals wounds, sores and phlegm disorders.

With regard to all the above meats the upper half of the body is heavier in male animals and the lower half of the body is heavier in females, whilst the flesh of pregnant animals is heavy throughout and that of female quadrupeds is light. In the case of birds the flesh of the male is always lighter. The head, shoulders, chest, back, hips and waist are in ascending order of heaviness; similarly with regard to the seven bodily constituents [nutriment, blood, flesh, fat, bone, marrow, semen] each successive one is heavier.

Fresh meat [one or two months old] has cool power, whilst old meat [three or more months old] is warm and nutritious. One-year-old meat is especially effective in subduing wind imbalances and it increases digestive heat, whereas raw, frozen or burned meat is heavy and hard to digest. On the other hand dried and cooked meats are light in power and easy to digest.

Oils

Oils include butter, sesame oil, marrow and fat, each in turn heavier than the previous one. They have a sweet taste and cool, aperient and oily powers, with blunt, thin, pliable and moist secondary qualities. Oils are recommended [as beneficial] for the aged, for children, in debility, emaciation, coarse complexion, semen deficiency, leucorrhoea, following purgation, mental strain, and whenever there is the threat of a wind disorder.

Fresh butter has cool power, increases semen, improves the complexion and eliminates bile fever. Old butter [nine or more months] is effective for mental disturbance, loss of memory and fainting [and for wounds]. Clarified ghee sharpens the mind, lends clarity to the memory and increases the heat and strength of the body. It also increases one's lifespan and has the power to perform thousands of [beneficial] functions.

Water on the surface of curd, cheese from the thick milk of a cow that has just calved, and dried cheese all improve appetite and cure mild constipation and phlegm imbalances. Residual butter [from churns, etc.] eliminates phlegm-wind combinations and increases digestive heat. Similarly butter of sheep and of the she-yak dispel cold and wind disorders. The butter of the dzo is of balanced, cool and warm power. The cooling butter of cow and goat eliminates wind fevers.

Sesame oil, with its hot and sharp powers, puts flesh on under-weight people and slims down those who are over-weight. In either case it toughens the body and eradicates phlegm-wind combinations.

Mustard oil subdues wind imbalances and increases phlegm and bile, whilst marrow grease dispels wind disorders and increases the power of semen and phlegm.

Fats cure aches in the joints, burns, wind imbalances and disorders of the ears, brain and womb. Those who rely on oils will find that they stimulate digestive heat, act as internal cleansers, spontaneously fortify the bodily constituents and enhance the strength and complexion. They also sustain the sense organs, provide vigor in old age and enable one to live for a hundred years as the Great Sage has affirmed.

Vegetables

Vegetables include garlic and onion, which are hot (-tasting), and dandelion and *Picris hieracioides,* which are bitter. They grow either in dry or damp areas and are (specifically) of dry, moist, prepared and raw types. The dry types have a warm, light power that eliminates cold disorders and the moist types have cool and heavy power, whereby fever may be eliminated.

Spring onions increase sleep, sharpen the appetite and eliminate combined phlegm and wind disorders. Garlic is heavy and cool, has an anthelmintic action and eradicates wind fever. Fresh radish has a light, warm power and increases digestive heat. One-year-old radish has heavy, cool powers and increases phlegm. Turnip has the same powers as radish and protects one from all types of poisoning. Hill garlic of all types is hard to digest, improves the appetite and has heavy power. *Rheum emodi* and *chu.lo* eliminate phlegm disorders and improve the appetite. (Partaking of) any (such) vegetables closes the mouths of the channels and weakens the power of medicines.

Prepared Foods

Regarding the section on prepared foods: rice porridge of thin, medium and thick consistencies and cooked rice are in descending order of lightness. Thin rice porridge quenches the thirst, prevents emaciation and dispels the remnants of disease (e.g., following purgation). It also normalizes the digestion, balances the bodily constituents, increases the digestive heat and renders the channels flexible. Rice porridge of medium consistency increases the digestive heat, satisfies hunger and thirst and cures debility, wasting diseases, digestive disorders and constipation. Thick rice porridge stops diarrhoea, improves the appetite and quenches the thirst. These [three types of] rice porridge are recommended in weakness and debility following (any form of) purgation. Well cooked rice, boiled with spices (longpeper, ginger, etc.) becomes light in power and easy to digest, whereas cooked rice boiled with meat broth or milk takes on a heavy power. Roasted rice stops diarrhoea and unites fractures. With regard to cereal broths, barley broth constipates and reduces the digestive heat. [Lightly cooked] roasted grain(-broth) is light and smooth and readily digestible. Roasted grain flour, when uncooked, acts as a tonic and has heavy power, but when cooked [as dumplings] it becomes light, smooth and easy to digest.

(When any of the above foods are) stale they reduce the digestive heat. Paste of roasted grain flour is easy to digest, deprives one of strength and cures disorders of all three humors. Dumpling (of roasted flour wine) cures wind disorders and facilitates digestion, whilst the sour [clear part of this wine] improves the appetite and cures imbalances of (all) the (three) humors. The residual part of the wine (in the bottom of the vessel) has no beneficial qualities.

Meat soup provides strength, satisfies and is beneficial in wind disorders. Broth of dried dough is supremely recommended for wind disorders. Nettle stew cures wind disorders, increases digestive heat and raises phlegm and bile. Stew of mallow and *Plantago depressa* increases digestive heat and stops diarrhoea. Stew of *Typhonium giganteum* cures wind disorders, dries wounds and increases phlegm and bile. (*sne*)[5] chenopodium stew is harmful to the eyes and removes flatulence. Red Mon (*sne*)[6] *Chenopodium aristatum* stew cures disorders of all three humors. Stew of gray and yellow dandelion has cool power and cures fevers, whilst stew of *Cremanthodium* cures heat disorders, bile fevers and headaches. Thick pea soup improves the appetite, increases phlegm and wind, absorbs body oil and eliminates undigested seed oil.

Fresh leaf stew has balanced [hot and cold power], whilst cooked withered leaves increase phlegm and wind. Stew of mustard leaves causes disturbance in the phlegm and bile, whilst stew of Angelica and *Polygonatum cirrifolium* cures phlegm and wind (disorders). Radish stew increases digestive heat and stops diarrhoea, whereas stew of garlic and (wild) hill garlic is beneficial in wind disorders.

Salt enhances the flavor of all kinds of food, increases digestive heat, facilitates digestion and regularizes bowel movement. *Zanthoxylum* opens the mouths of the channels and increases phlegm and wind. Ginger increases (digestive) heat and Asafoetida cures wind disorders. Spices in general improve the flavor of all foods and stimulate the appetite.

BEVERAGES

These include milk, water and alcohol among others. Milk opposes wind, water opposes bile and alcohol opposes phlegm, whereas milk increases phlegm, water increases wind, and alcohol increases bile.

Milk

Almost all types of milk have a sweet (natural) taste and (post-) digestive taste and by their greasy, heavy power increase the bodily constituents as well as brighten the complexion and eliminate wind and bile. Milk increases virility and phlegm, and has cool and heavy powers.

Cow's milk is beneficial for punctured lung and consumption; it heals chronic infectious fever and frequent urination, and dispels lethargy. Goat's milk cures asthmatic conditions and sheep's milk cures wind disorders but is harmful for the heart. She-yak's milk is harmful in phlegm and bile disorders, whilst the milk of horse and donkey heals lung diseases but increases (mental) dullness. Cold milk has heavy and cool powers and increases bacteria and phlegm, whereas if it is boiled it is light and warm in power. Condensed milk is heavy and indigestible whereas lukewarm milk [fresh from the cow] is similar to nectar in qualities.

After the essence (butter) has been extracted from the milk the whey that remains cures (infectious fever) imbalances, influenza, scattered fever, disturbed fever and diarrhoea.

All curds have a sour (natural) taste and post-digestive taste, cool and greasy power, dispel dry stools and wind fever, and improve the appetite. Fresh whey is astringent, sour, and light in power, increases digestive heat and removes tumors, spleen disorders, hemorrhoids and undigested butter. The surface water from the curd loosens the bowels, makes the stool thinner and cleanses the interior of the channels. The residual water from cheese does not increase wind or bile but it eliminates phlegm. Cooked curd removes flatulence and diarrhoea accompanied by fever.

The dairy products of sheep and of the she-yak have warm and highly nutritious power, whilst those of the cow and goat are cool and light. Dairy products obtained from the dzo have balanced (warm and cool) powers.

Water

[The different types of] water include rainwater, melted snow, river water, spring water, well water, sea and forest water. Rainwater is of supreme quality and the rest are successively inferior. Rain water is of indeterminate but pleasant taste, is invigorating and satisfying, has cool, light power and is like nectar. Melted snow water comes in rushing torrents. It is very fine, cool water which is hard for the digestive power to withstand. Still calm areas of water produce germs, elephantiasis, and heart diseases. Good water is that which comes from a clean area and which has felt the touch of the sun and wind. Muddy or marshy water which contains algae, grass, leaves or trees, or which is in the shade of these, or water which is contaminated by salt, insects or effluence, will increase all three humors.

Cool water cures fainting, fatigue, hangovers, vertigo, vomiting, thirst, obesity, blood and bile disorders and poisoning. Freshly boiled water increases digestive heat, facilitates digestion, cures hiccoughs, promptly cures distension of the abdomen caused by phlegm, cures asthmatic conditions, fresh colds and infectious fevers. Cool boiled water does not increase phlegm and cures bile conditions, but if it is left standing for one day (or more) it acquires toxic properties and increases all three humors.

Alcohols

Liquors have sweet, sour and bitter tastes with a sour post-digestive taste, and sharp, warm, coarse, thin and mildly aperient powers. They generate heat, increase self-confidence, induce sleep and cure phlegm and wind (disorders).

Drinking to excess transforms the mind, making one reckless and removes one's sense of shame. In the first stage of intoxication one maintains a reckless state, ceases to consider the opinions of others and feels comfortable and at ease. In the second stage one is like a crazed elephant and commits transgressions of moral discipline whilst in the final (third) stage one lies unconscious like a corpse, unperceiving and oblivious.

Fresh liquor is heavy in power, whilst matured alcohol is light and that of medium age increases digestive heat and facilitates digestion. Barley beer, rice beer and wheat beer are in ascending order of heaviness whilst beer of thick-shelled barley, sixty-day barley and roasted grain are each lighter in turn. Hot [tasting matured liquor] cures disorders of blood, bile and phlegm.

This concludes the sixteenth chapter, on the principles of diet, from *The Quintessence Tantra, the Secret Oral Tradition of the Eight Branches of the Science of Healing.*

17. Principles of Diet: Dietary Restrictions

Then the Sage Rig.pahi.ye.she spoke these words: O Great Sage, listen. Food and drink entail certain restraints, namely on poisonous and unwholesome foods which snatch away one's life and imbalance the humors. These are to be guarded against. [For example] in the Royal Palace is retained a life-sustaining healer-preceptor to [relieve] the King of [the risk of] poisoning by food or drink.

Poisonous food has an unusual color, odor and taste, and when it is burned the smoke takes on the hue of a peacock's neck. [At the same time] the tongues of flame will swirl to one side and sparks will fly out [a long way]. If [such poisonous food] is seen by a crow it will caw [loudly], whereas a peacock will be pleased. If it is given to a dog its stomach will become hot, with vomiting as the result.

Meat containing poison will be red, a (hot) iron will not adhere to it or it will swell. [The steam from such] prepared meat or from meat [dipped] in liquor will irritate the eyes and cause them to smart.

One who has administered poison experiences a dry mouth, perspires, trembles with fear, is restless and looks in [all] directions with guilt and apprehension. Having understood [the above] one should henceforth refrain from giving harm to others.

Eating unwholesome food is akin to ingesting compounded poison. Partaking of curd that has not set together with fresh liquor [for example, grain beer] is unwholesome, as is (the combination of) fish with milk. [It is similarly] unwholesome [to combine] milk with fruit, or birds' eggs with fish; cooked pulses with cane sugar and curd is [an unwholesome combination], as is frying mushrooms in mustard oil. It would also be unwholesome to partake of chicken mixed with curd or of an even [combination of] honey and (seed) oil. [Similarly unwholesome] is fresh butter kept in a bronze vessel for ten days.

It is unwholesome to eat (lion's) meat roasted on a fire of barberry (wood) and to partake of mushrooms after eating (powdered) calcite. [An unwholesome combination would be] meat that has been mixed with or has even come into contact with a white [dairy product], sour [liquor] or roasted grain flour. Similarly unwholesome would be either food steamed shut and left for seven days, or a combination of milk with anything sour.

Fresh intake of food when the previous meal is still undigested and [other] unwholesome food (combinations) cause an adverse reaction. Intake of food to which one is not accustomed or untimely dining leads to poisoning. One who takes (regular) exercise, sustained by oil [ghee, etc.], having great digestive heat, being in the prime of youth with strong body, and who is (to some degree) accustomed to such foods will not be (adversely) affected (by them). If one wishes to rely on a (formerly) unwholesome food, or give up a wholesome one, one should accustom oneself by introducing [ever increasing or decreasing] portions [to one's diet]. By abruptly giving up [a certain food], or by introducing [a new food], the humors will quickly become imbalanced.

The wise will avoid [foods which are] non-beneficial and harmful to the body, the latter being a combination of 'harmers' [the humors] and objects of harm (the bodily constituents and excretions).

This concludes the seventeenth chapter, on dietary restrictions, from *The Quintessence Tantra, the Secret Oral Tradition of the Eight Branches of the Science of Healing.*

18. Principles of Diet: The Correct Amount of Food

Then the Sage Rig.pahi.ye.she spoke these words: O Great Sage, listen. At all times eat the correct amount of food. [The powers of] foods may be inferred from their degree of heaviness or lightness. If the food is light [-powered] one fills the stomach, (whereas) if the food is heavy (-powered) one should only half fill the stomach. From this explanation one realizes that [the food] will be digested with ease and comfort. Such [a principle] will promote longevity and increase the digestive heat.

If one consumes only a small amount of food this will not enhance one's complexion nor strength but will give rise to all wind disorders. If one overeats indigestion [will result] and mucus will increase, blocking [the function of] the firelike equalizing wind in the duodenum. The digestive heat will deteriorate and all the humors will be increased. Therefore one should combine the food and the digestive heat. One should fill two parts of the stomach with food, one with drink, and in the fourth part leave room for the [firelike equalizing] wind, [the decomposing phlegm and the digestive bile].

After eating one should drink (enough) to satisfy and [enable the nutriment] to pervade (the body), as this decomposes the food, facilitates digestion, develops the body and increases strength. [However drinking] is harmful for [those suffering from] hoarseness, punctured lung, [excess throat] mucus, (common) cold, and diseases above the neck.

If one's digestive heat is weak, after eating meat one should take alcohol, (whereas) in distension of the stomach due to indigestion one should drink [hot] boiled water after meals. A thin person [wishing] to put on weight should take alcohol, whilst an overweight person should drink honey in water in order to lose weight. One who ingests curd, liquor, food contaminated by poison or honey will afterwards derive benefit from drinking cool water. (According to) whether one drinks during, at the end of or at the beginning of one's meals one will become respectively of medium build, overweight or thin.

The humors will not follow the wrong paths, the digestive heat will flourish, the body will become light, the appetite will be healthy, the sense organs will become clear, one's strength will increase and stool, urine and gas will be expelled without difficulty: (all these advantages) will arise from having adhered to a balanced diet.

This concludes the eighteenth chapter, on dietary restrictions and balanced diet, from *The Quintessence Tantra, the Secret Oral Tradition of the Eight Branches of the Science of Healing*.

19. Principles of Medicine: Tastes and Post-Digestive Tastes

Then the sage Yid.las.skyes asked: O Master, Sage Rig.pahi.ye.she, how may we learn about the principles of compounding medicines? We request the Physician, the Sovereign Healer, to explain!

At this the Teacher replied: O Great Sage, listen. (The) instruction in the principles of compounding medicines, which are the remedies for healing disease, is fourfold, (according to) (a) taste and (b) post-digestive taste (chapter nineteen), (c) power (chapter twenty) and (d) methods of compounding (chapter twenty-one).

TASTES OF MEDICINES

The first, taste, has five aspects, (namely,) (1) the basis (of taste), (2) divisions, (3) nature, (4) groups (of medicine having the same taste) and (5) the function (of taste).

The Basis and Divisions of Taste
   The basis [of taste] is derived from the five elements. The earth element provides a foundation (and) basis, the water element [provides] moisture, the fire element (generates) heat, the wind element [increases] movement and the space element affords room. Although the majority of medicines grow according to those factors they do not have the same taste. Earth and water [is sweet], fire and earth [is sour], water and fire [is salty], water

and wind [is bitter], fire and wind [is hot], earth and wind [is astringent]: from these (six) pairs the six tastes are produced.

The Natures of Taste

Earth-[natured] medicine has heavy, firm, blunt, smooth, greasy and dry (powers). Its function is to make (the limbs) firm, to develop (the body) and to make it compact, as well as to cure wind disorders.

Water-[natured] medicine has liquid, cool, heavy, blunt, oily and pliable powers. It provides moisture, softens the body, makes it compact and cures bile disorders.

Fire-[natured] medicine has hot, sharp, dry, coarse, light, oily and mobile powers. It increases (body) heat, matures (the bodily constituents), clears the complexion and cures phlegm disorders.

Wind-[natured] medicine has light, mobile, cold, coarse, absorbent and dry powers. It fortifies and articulates the body, spreads [nutriments and so forth throughout the body] and cures phlegm and bile disorders.

(The) space [element] is common to and pervades [the other] four elements and [all] medicines. Its function is to bestow hollowness, to provide extensive space and to cure disorders arising from a combination of [all three humors]. Therefore, whether it is natural or has been incorporated into a compound, there is nothing on the surface of the earth that is not a medicine.

Medicine having ascending force has the qualities of fire and wind, (whereas) the power of medicine with descending force arises from (the) earth and water (elements). The [power of] purgative medicines largely arises from the first of the tastes (i.e., sweet). The [six] tastes are sweet, sour, salty, bitter, hot and astringent. In this order (of six tastes) each one is more powerful as a healing agent than the one that follows it. By nature taste is said to be that which is distinguished by the tongue. Thus when a sweet taste is experienced it sticks to the tongue and, being tasty, it produces craving. A sour taste sets the teeth on edge, puckers the face and [causes] one's month to water. Saltiness is heating and is a sialagogue, whilst a bitter taste purifies the mouth odor and depresses the appetite. A hot taste burns the tongue and mouth and causes the eyes to water, whereas an astringent taste sticks to the palate, producing a coarse sensation.

Groups of Medicines Having the Same Taste

[Six groups of medicines are enumerated according to each individual taste.] The group of medicines having sweet taste includes liquorice, raisins, saffron, bamboo concretion, cassia pods, *Polygonatum cirrifolium, Asparagus racemosus,* Angelica, sugar-candy, raw cane sugar (jaggery), honey, meat, butter and the like.

The group of medicines having sour taste includes pomegranate, sea buckthorn *(Hippophae rhamnoides), Chaenomeles tibetica,* emblic myrobalan, Indian juniper, *Schizandra sphaerandra,* curd, whey and curd 'culture', grain beer, etc.

The group of medicines having salty taste includes rock salt, wood salt, horn salt, black 'sanchal' salt, white mineral salt, mirabilite, soda salt (saltpetre), white rock salt, ash salt, aragonite (Tartar salt) and salsoda (sodium bicarbonate).

The group of medicines having bitter taste includes neem, Indian gentian, *Aconitum balfouri, Picrorhiza kurroa,* bitter cucumber, Conessi (Kurchi), musk, (animal) bile, Indian barberry, Malabar nut tree, mineral exudate, *Gentiana straminea, Corydalis edulis,* etc.

The group of medicines having hot taste includes black pepper, wild ginger, longpeper, fresh (moist) ginger, Asafoetida, a type of *Anemone rivularis (srub.ka), che.tsha, Arisaema intermedium,* onion, garlic, etc.

The group of medicines having astringent taste includes (white) sandalwood, chebulic myrobalan, beleric myrobalan, blue Utpala flower *(Nelumbo nucifera),* meadow cranesbill, powdered (pine)-root *(Padus asiatica),* acorns and Tibetan tamarisk.

Camphor and wild rhubarb, etc., have a combination of tastes, and from these one can research similar [examples of taste combination]. [Camphor is said to have a primary bitter taste with a threefold combination of bitter, hot and astringent. Wild rhubarb is said to have sour, sweet and astringent tastes combined.]

Exposition of the Function of Tastes in Curing Diseases

Sweet, sour, salty and hot tastes dispel wind disorders. Bitter, sweet and astringent tastes cure bile disorders, whilst hot, sour, and salty tastes cure phlegm ailments.

[The function of] sweet taste in particular is wholesome, it increases the strength and the bodily constituents, and is beneficial for the aged, for children, for the undernourished, in hoarseness and for [punctured] lungs. It develops the body, heals wounds, brightens the complexion, and clears the sense organs. Sweet taste promotes longevity, sustains the body and cures poisoning and combined disorders of wind and bile. Partaking (of sweet things) in excess increases phlegm and fat, reduces the digestive heat and produces (fleshy) excrescences, urinary disorders, goiter and glandular growths.

Sour-tasting substances increase heat, improve the appetite, satisfy [the mind], break down [food], remove [phlegm imbalances], and facilitate digestion; external application of sour substances causes loss of sensation and moves blocked wind. Partaking of sour things in excess increases blood and bile, makes the body limp, and produces blurred vision, dizziness, first and second stages of oedema, erysipelas, cutaneous itch, pimples, thirst and contagious fevers.

Salty taste toughens the body and removes whorls (of wind, etc.) and blockages [of the channels, etc.]. [Hot salt] fomentation increases perspiration and digestive heat and improves the appetite. Partaking [of salty things] in excess causes falling hair and greying of the hair, increases wrinkles, decreases strength and produces thirst, leprosy, erysipelas and blood and bile disorders.

Bitter taste cures anorexia, worms, thirst, poisoning, leprosy, fainting, infectious fevers, [vomiting of] fluid and bile disorders. It dries necrosis, fat, grease, marrow, stool and urine. [Bitter taste also improves] mental alertness and cures breast disorders and hoarseness, Partaking [of bitter things] in excess consumes the bodily constituents and increases wind and phlegm.

Hot taste cures throat disorders, [throat] constriction, leprosy and second stage oedema. It dries wounds, increases [digestive] heat, facilitates digestion and improves appetite. [Hot taste also] dries fat and necrosis, [acts as a] purgative and opens the channels. Partaking [of hot tasting things] in excess consumes the semen and strength of the body, causes physical deformity, shivering, fainting and pain in the waist, back, etc.

Astringent taste dries blood, bile, fat and necrosis, heals

wounds, cleans fat and brightens the complexion. Partaking [of astringent tasting things] in excess collects mucus, retains stool, causes distension of the abdomen and heart disorders, dries [nutriment, fluid, etc.] and constricts the mouths of the channels.

In summary, sweet taste cures wind and bile [disorders] and also, with the exception of old barley and the meat of dry land animals, it mostly increases phlegm. Wild yak meat, fish, mutton and honey are beneficial [in phlegm disorders]. Sour taste cures phlegm and also increases bile. (However) sour emblic myrobalan cures blood and bile diseases and fever. Salty taste cures wind and phlegm (disorders) and, with the exceptions of wood salt and rock salt, increases bile. Excess intake [of these two exceptions] with their heavy power, increases phlegm. Bitter taste cures bile and also increases phlegm-wind. (However) Indian beech and Heart-leaved moonseed cure phlegm-wind [combined]. Hot [taste] cures wind and phlegm and, except for garlic and longpeper, increases bile. Excess [intake of hot tasting things with their] light, coarse [power] also increases wind. Astringent taste cures bile and, with the exceptions of chebulic myrobalan and beleric myrobalan, mostly arouses both phlegm and wind.

POST-DIGESTIVE TASTES

After ingestion [the medicine] meets the digestive heat and is then digested by the [decomposing] phlegm, the [digestive] bile and the [firelike equalizing] wind in turn. Sweet and salty tastes become sweet in the post-digestive phase. Sour things retain the same taste, and the three tastes of bitter, hot and astringent become bitter. Each [post-digestive] taste cures two of the three humors: [sweet post-digestive taste cures wind and bile, sour post-digestive taste cures phlegm and wind, bitter post-digestive taste cures phlegm and bile].

Thus it was said. This concludes the nineteenth chapter, on the exposition of tastes and post-digestive tastes, from *The Quintessence Tantra, the Secret Oral Tradition of the Eight Branches of the Science of Healing.*

20. The Principles of Medicines: Powers of Medicines

Then sage Rig.pahi.ye.she spoke these words: O Great Sage, listen. The power of medicines is twofold: (a) the power of taste and (b) the natural power [of the substance]. This has been taught according to general and specific sections.

GENERAL SECTION

First the powers, strength and [secondary] qualities of all three [humors] are explained. The eight powers are heavy, oily, cool, blunt, light, coarse, hot and sharp. The first four cure wind and bile [i.e., heavy and oily cure wind, and cool and blunt cure bile]. The last four powers cure phlegm. The three powers light, coarse and cool increase wind, whilst hot, sharp and oily [all] increase bile. The four powers heavy, oily, cool and blunt increase phlegm. These eight powers are all the essence of the [secondary] qualities and, since they are endowed with exceptional powers they are called 'forces'. *Gang.chen*[1] and *hBigs. byed*[2] are respectively endowed with the strength of the moon and sun with their cool and warm [natures] and so these are called 'strengths'.

Hot powered [medicines] cure cold disorders and cool powered [medicines] cure hot diseases.

The twenty characteristics [of disease] are subdued by the seventeen [secondary] qualities, namely: smoothness, heaviness, warmth, oiliness, firmness, coldness, bluntness, coolness, pliability, fluidity, dryness, absorbency, heat, lightness, sharpness, coarseness and motility. Therefore the [secondary] qualities thus explained mostly derive from the [six] tastes. The tastes [in turn] depend on the earth [and the rest of the five elements].

[The powers of] heaviness, oiliness, etc., arise from [the tastes]. The three different [tastes] salty, astringent and sweet are [each] heavier in turn. Similarly salty, sour and sweet are [each] oilier [in turn, whilst] astringent, bitter and sweet are [each] cooler [in turn, whilst], bitter, astringent and sweet are [each more] blunt [in turn]. The three different [tastes] sour, hot and bitter are in turn more light and coarse, whereas the three respective [tastes] hot, sour and salty are in turn more hot and sharp.

[Generally if the tastes, etc., of any substances] are not refined they will be [most] powerful. If the tastes and powers [etc.] are equal the individual basis [elements which form the power can vary in their ratio] and change the strength [of the medicine]. By force of compounding [variations in the strength of the medicines] will arise and if the compounding is unbalanced the [taste] will outweigh the digestive taste, [and thus the power of the medicine will be neutralized]. [If] all the ingredients are compounded in a balanced [way, the medicine will be effective by virtue of] its taste. Taste itself will not be harmful to the condition [in cases where the medicine] works by virtue of its post-digestive taste. [For example: the normally hot powered wood salt cures rather than harms a bile disorder by virtue of its sweet post-digestive taste]. [In other cases the medicine] will work by virtue of its power even when this is opposite to the taste. [For example: bitter Indian beech, instead of increasing wind and phlegm, cures wind and phlegm conditions with its warm power.] [Therefore] compounding should be done by combining [ingredients which work by] taste with those which work according to power or post-digestive taste.

SPECIFIC SECTION

(The) exposition of the powers of individual natural sub-

stances (has) eight sections:
(1) precious [metal] medicines
(2) stone medicines
(3) earth medicines
(4) tree medicines
(5) resins
(6) plants
(7) herbs
(8) animal products

(1) The Powers of Precious [Metals]

Gold: [gold has thirty-two names and is of two types—red and yellow. It is said that gold from the hDzambu River was eaten by the Me.zan[3] which deposited it in its droppings in China and Hor.[4] From this red gold the local people used to make very sweet sounding bells. Another type of red gold, called *dzhye. khyim,* resembles rust red copper. If a solution of aconite is applied to it, it takes on a rainbow hue and thus is a most excellent test for poison. Yellow gold is also of two types — superior and ordinary. The superior type is in the form of unwrought gold, whilst the common type is yellow with a reddish hue. Other types have a bluish hue or are very pale. By way of determining whether a sample is gold or not, artificial gold has astringent taste and cool digestive power. The *Eight Branches* text states: "Just as water does not adhere to the petals of a lotus, so ingestion of gold will prevent poison from adhering to the limbs."] Gold promotes longevity, strengthens the aged, acts as an antidote to gem poisoning [and dispels spirits and nagas[5]].

Silver: [silver has ten names and is known to be smelted from ore. It is of two types—'goat silver' and 'sheep silver.' However, nowadays Hor silver is called silver *kha,* Chinese silver is called *ona kha,* Indian silver is called *ba,* Mon silver is called *tram kha,* and Russian silver is called *dra men.* These are all 'goat silvers.' Kham silver is called *zho.kha.ma.* The silver which comes from iron, tin, lead and copper, etc., is 'sheep silver.' Silver can also be extracted from wood and earth. It has the same (astringent) taste and post-digestive taste as gold, and by its power] it dries lymph disorders, pus and blood.

Copper: [copper has twelve names and the superior type is of natural origin. So-called iron copper is dark red, rough and smelted, whereas 'gold copper' is red and pliable. These and other types have sweet taste and post-digestive taste and cool power.] Copper dries pus and cures fevers of the lungs and liver.

Iron: [iron has nine names and comes from iron-ore, lodestone, *mdung.rtse* rock[6] and from animals. It may be black or white and is of four types. Also iron has sour taste and cool power, whereby] it cures liver poisoning, eye diseases and first stage oedema.

Herewith is concluded the section on metals which can be melted.

Turquoise: [turquoise is of two types, superior and ordinary. Of the superior types *drug.dkar* is pale blue and very bright, whilst *drug.dmar* is bright reddish-blue and greasy. The third, *g-yu.spyang,* is brighter than the first two sub-types. Among the ordinary types *bar.g-yu* resembles *drug.dmar* and *g-yu.sngon* resembles *drug.dkar.* A Chinese turquoise also exists.] Turquoise cures poison-fever and liver-fever.

Pearl: [pearl has seven names. The first type, *rakta mutika,* is held to be supremely precious, because Buddhas have manifested as the red creature from which red pearl is obtained. The second type, *gandza mu.tig,* is sparkling white and comes from inside the skull or tusk of elephant. The third type of pearl is Wa.lu.mu.tig, which is bright blue and comes from South India. It is found inside the leaves of the *du.ya* tree after the rain has fallen. The fourth type, *ram.pa.mu.tig,* is slightly greenish and is the size of a pea. In East India it is found in the leaves of the banana tree after rain has fallen. The fifth type, *smad.mu.tig,* is bright red and comes from the West of Hor, where it is found in the brain of a species of snake.

The sixth type of pearl, *shing.pi.ka.mu.tig,* varies in size and has a pale yellow radiance. It comes from the stomach of a sea creature called *spang.rtsi,* which resembles an oyster and is found around Sri Lanka.

All types of pearls without eyes are of male gender and those having many layers are considered female. Pearl] prevents loss of cerebral fluid and cures all types of poisoning.

Mother of Pearl has three names and its power is not unlike that of pearl.

Conch shell: [conch shell has five names and is of superior and ordinary types. The superior type, *g-yas.bkhyil* (lit., 'right clockwise swirl'), incarnates five times as a conch and is lily white, with a clockwise swirl. Another superior type, *gzi.dung*, is red in color. The ordinary types are recognized as having an anti-clockwise swirl, and there is also a 'thorny' conch, *tsher.ma.chan.* All four types] dry pus, puncture whorls [of pus, etc.], cure bone fever [and are beneficial for the eyes].

Coral: coral [has three names and is a type of tree which grows by the sea in rock and sand. The *Vajra Dakini* text and others state that it is known to be red tipped with a white root; a black type also exists. The red coral] cures liver fever, channel fever and fever from poisoning.

Lapis Lazuli: Lapis Lazuli [has four names and is a type of blue stone. The gold flecked type is called 'gold lapis,' whilst the plain type is 'stone lapis.' Both types] cure poisoning, lymph disorders and leprosy.

2.   The Powers of Stone Medicines
smug.po.sbal.rgyab (lit. 'the brown frog's back stone'): **Hematite**: is of two types, The 'male frog' [type is brown, hard, heavy and similar to a frog's back. The superior type bears a stupa design and has large bumps, whilst the common type has small bumps only. The superior quality of] the 'female frog' [type bears a lotus design and has no bumps, whilst the common type is just without bumps. Both types] expel, extract and dry lymph, maintain bone resin, heal fractures and sustain the brain.

dkar.po.sbal.rgyab (lit. 'the white frog's back stone'): **Stalactite:** Hematite: Is similar to white *chhig.thub* (white pyrolusite) and brown *chhig.thub* (brown pyrolusite). [It is hard, heavy and pointed. The male type bears a stupa design, whilst the female type has a lotus design. These correspond in quality to the two types of brown stone above. With regard to white and brown pyrolusite, the superior type is ice-like, soft, pointed and breaks into needle-like pieces. Some people used to call the brown type 'stone camphor' because of its strong odor. It is dark brown and shaped like slate]. The white type has the same powers as the brown 'frog's back' stone.

gangs.thig (lit. 'drop of snow'): **Smithsonite:** Calamine: [One type of Smithsonite is a female type of quartz, white in color. It is spongy, flexible and soft. Another type is found in hard, white globules the size of a pea.] Both types cure liver fever.

khab.len: **Lodestone:** Magnetic Ore: [This has four names and also is of four types: *hgugs.byed, gchod.byed, hbigs.byed* and *skor.byed.* It is of superior, medium and ordinary qualities. The superior type is found to the south of Mount Meru, where there is a lion shaped rock of lodestone. Therefore the needle of the compass points north. Medium quality lodestone comes from China and can hold ten needles together in a chain. The ordinary type is dark brown and can attract needles.] Lodestone expels arrowheads [bullets, shrapnel, etc.] through the digestive tract and cures disorders of the brain, bones and channels.

be.snabs: **Yellow Halloysite:** [is of two types: pale yellow and yellowish brown.] It cures fractures and glandular growths, and stimulates flesh growth.

man(y)jira: **Fossil Muscovite:** Ophicalcite: [Zur.mkhar[7] asserts this to be a hard black stone required to retain mercury (during processing), whereas Gong.smanpa and sKyem.ts(h)e.dwang[8] assert it to be a shiny liver-colored stone. It has no fixed color and bears the design of the horn of a goat or sheep. The male type is coarse and the female type is smooth. The medium types are regarded as natural. All types of] muscovite cure bone fevers.

phag.mgo: **Pig's Head Fossil:** [bears the shape of a pig's head and is orange in color]. It heals bone disorders and drains lymph [accumulations].

bye.mgo: **Sparrow's Head Fossil:** *Spiriferoides: Cyrtiospirifer sinensis:* [The superior type is light blue, smooth and small. The ordinary type is pale red, large, coarse and resembles a hawk's head. Both types] promote flesh growth.

gser.rdo: **Gold Ore:** [has three names. Here it is called by two names: *byang.khog* and *mig.nad.dus.kyi.pa.bya.* It is of indeterminate shape and is brown and yellow; when broken the interior has a golden sheen.]

dngul.rdo: **Silver Ore:** [has three names and is of (indeterminate) shape. It is brown externally and has a shiny silver hue on the inside. Silver is obtained by smelting it]. Both of the above types of ore drain lymph [accumulations].

stang.zil: **Massicotite:** [has four names and is a black stone which breaks into sparkling needle-like pieces. It is so dark in color that it is said to resemble the hair of the Lord Buddha].

gser.zil: **Vermiculite:** Litharge: Mineral Oxide of Lead: [resembles gold ore and has various shapes. It is a soft stone which breaks into long, sparkling needle-like pieces].

dngul.zil: **Mineral Sulphate of Calcium:** Carbonate of Lime: [varies in shape and is softer than silver ore. It has a greenish hue and breaks into needle-like pieces. All three types of zil] remove discoloration of the bone.

gru.bzhi (lit. 'square stone'): type of **Pyrite**, e.g., of Galena or Analcite: [has seven names (*pha.wang.long.bug, pha.wang.chho.long,* etc.): It is of two types: black and white, and yellow and brown. The white or yellow types are beneficial for the eyes and the black or brown ones are beneficial against rabies poisoning. Its general power is to] heal brain disorders and to drain lymph [accumulations].

chog.la.ma or *rgya.mtshal:* **Cinnabar:** [is of two types: red and white. Apart from the naturally formed type it is also prepared artificially from silver orpiment. The dark red type fragments into sparkling needle-like pieces. Both types] maintain the channels and the bone resin. (The white type cures smallpox fever.)

rdo.klad (lit. 'stone brain'): **Halloysite:** [is a white 'pimply' stone that looks like a brain]. It maintains the brain and stimulates flesh growth.

li.gris: **Red Lead:** Minium: [has six names. One coarse type is obtained from stone whilst a smooth type comes from earth, and a sticky type is obtained from wood. In Nepal an artificial type is made from lead. All types of red lead] stop necrosis.

rdo.chhu (lit. 'stone water'): A type of **Actinolite:** [has two names and bears a rippling design. It is found around hot springs. The Malaya commentary states that the white type is called *rdo.rgyus* (lit. 'stone tendon') whilst the blue type is called *mthing.rgyus* (lit. 'indigo tendon') or Actinolite asbestos. The yellow type] heals fractures.

rdo.mkhris: **Yellow Ochre:** Argile glauconicus: [The superior type has a yellow bile color and is of uncertain shape. It sticks to the tongue and has a slightly bitter taste. The common type is bitter and of uncertain color. Both types] constrict the mouths of the channels.

bshah.dkar: **Stannic Ore:** [is mixed with copper to make bell metal and in its natural state looks like silver ore. It] promotes flesh growth.

ldong.ros: **Realgar:** Red Orpiment: [has three names and is an orange mineral with (its own peculiar) odor.]

ba.bla: **Yellow Orpiment:** Arsenolite: [has four names and is of a paler, yellower hue than the red type with its own (peculiar) odor. Both types of orpiment] arrest malignant glandular growths and necrosis [and protect from infectious fever caused by spirits].

rdo.sol: **Coal:** [has a black color similar to charcoal and is used as such. It] dissolves stones [gall stones, kidney stones, etc.] and constricts the mouths of the channels.

ba.nu: **Carbonate of Chalk:** [is a stone shaped like a cow's udder and is of uncertain color. When broken it smells like burnt horn. It is of smooth and coarse types, corresponding to male and female types, with a (transitional) neuter type.]

rdo.rgyus (lit. 'stone tendon'): **Actinolite:** Stibine: A smooth, white stone with the texture of a tendon. The blue type is called *mthing.rgyus* (lit: 'indigo tendon') and the green type is called *spang.rgyus* (lit. 'meadow tendon'). Carbonate of chalk and the three types of actinolite heal [disorders of] the ligaments [and tendons].

ti.ts(h)e: **Galenite:** [This stone may be smelted to produce lead. The superior type is yellow and the common type is red. It] heals wounds and is beneficial in eye diseases and 'body odor'.

mtshal: **Chinese Vermilion:** [This refers to mercuric sulphide ore or cinnabar. It has eight names and varies in color but is mostly black. It] heals wounds and cures fevers of the lungs, liver and channels.

lig.bu.mig: **Malachite:** Skt. *potanchala:* [has two names and, according to Zur.mkhar, is a type of *stang.zil* (see above). Others maintain that it is a heavier type of *mdung.rtse,* or a brown *mdung.rtse.* The *Pad.dkar.chhun.po* (Bouquet of White Lotuses) text states, "Malachite is by nature a stone of orange, blue or green types, adorned with an eye. It is a precious stone obtained from water. It has the power to subdue harm (for example, epilepsy) from the (twenty-eight constellations of) moving stars." The supreme type has nine eyes and the superior type is hard, shiny and black with a white eye].

btsag: **Red Ochre:** Halloysite: [has two names and is found in the form of a red stone]. *yug* [is a blue type of Halloysite; red and blue Halloysite] cure eye diseases and bone fever and dry lymph [accumulations].

chong.zhi: **Calcite:** [has five names and is of five (major) types It] halts diarrhoea, cures phlegm fever [and is a principle ingredient of essence-extraction compounds].

rdo.thal (lit. 'stone ash'): **Limestone:** [is of many types and colors and is plentiful around hot springs. It is colloquially known as *rdo.zho* (lit. 'stone curd'). Burnt limestone disperses abdominal phlegm 'tumors'.]

ha.shig: **Talc:** [has four names (*thod.lo.kor,* etc.). It is white, red, blue, black or of uncertain color. Though it appears hard it is soft and one can draw on it]. It purges channel disorders.

mo.rdo (lit. 'female stone'): [For example, kidney- or gall-stones removed from the body of a woman. Such female stones] are beneficial for curing stone disorders [in men and vice versa. A certain similar smooth stone found on river banks is beneficial for blood clots and stone poisoning when used as a (cold) fomentation].

3. The Exposition of the Power of Earth Medicines

gser.gyis.bye.ma: **Golden Sand:** [has previously been (wrongly) identified as the small seeds of a tree or of a plant called *dwon.poi.rgyug.pa.* In actuality it is a sandlike substance obtained from the shores of lakes. The superior type is yellow. The common type is smoky colored, with bitter, hot taste. Nowadays it is found in abundance and so there is little chance of mistaking it. Both types] cure kidney disorders and urinary retention.

sindur: **Limonite:** Natural oxide of lead [has six names. The name 'sindur' means *ra.chhags* or blood, and it is asserted to be the menstrual blood of the dakinis.[9] It forms in caves and on the shores of lakes and is similar in color to red lead, i.e., reddish-yellow]. It heals channel fever and injuries in the vital organs. Limonite also dries pus and blood and is beneficial for burn wounds.

ze.tsha: **Saltpetre:** Mirabilite: [has four names and is found in caves and on old (clay) walls. It has a soft, oily texture and tastes like lake salt. The artificial type is white and crystal clear.

It] dissolves stones [for example in the kidneys, gall bladder, etc.], removes calculi and stone tumors [and dispels urinary retention].

ya.ba.ksha.ra: **Potash:** Aragonite: [The *hDod.hjor* commentary asserts that when calcinated blue barley is left overnight a saline formation, (potash) appears on the surface. An alternative translation is that *ya.ba* means barley and *ksha.ra* means transform. The *Zla.ba* text states that it is the ash of burnt barley, and, with regard to its power, the *Zla.zer* text states, "The burnt barley salt, *ya.ba.ka.ra,* cures tumors, heart disease and first stage oedema. These days it forms like white ash at the base of boulders and makes a crunching sound when squeezed in the hands. Thus there is little chance of confusing it with other salts."] It increases heat and purges tumors.

bul.tog: **Salsoda:** [has five names: *mdzi.bu.ka,* Tibetan salt, etc., and has a bitter taste similar to earth *ma.nu.* It is used in tea and so there is little chance of mistaking it.] It halts necrosis, digests [undigested roasted grain] flour [and cures poisoning].

mu.zi: **Sulphur:** [has sixteen names and is found around hot springs. It is of white, black and yellow types and the black one has two sub-types. Further details may be found in other texts. The superior type is yellow and the common type resembles amber. The white type which is mixed with earth often becomes yellow after processing. Yellow sulphur dispels spirits, and dries pus, blood, [lymph, etc.]. Black sulphur smells like horn and the best [black] type is shiny. The common black sulphur smells like burnt horn and cures erysipelas and contagious diseases].

nag.mtsur: **Black Alunite:** Vitriol: [has six names and is greenish-yellow. The bubbles of this mineral when boiled will turn copper red on contact, and, if sprinkled in a decoction of chebulic myrobalan, it will turn it black. [*ser.mtsur* (fibroferrite), the yellow type,] is used for dyeing wool and a solution of chebulic myrobalan will turn yellow when it is added. This and black alunite (*nag.mtsur*) halt necrosis, extract tumors [and are also beneficial for falling hair].

big.pan: **Chalcanthite:** Skt. *Nilathota:* [has similar qualities to mTsur and is blue. The whitish type is of two varieties and tastes, like *mtsur.* All types] remove small abscesses, disperse tumors, cure conjunctivitis [and alleviate wind fevers].

rdo.dreg (lit. 'stone dirt'): A type of **Lichen:** *Parmelia saxatilis:* [has thirteen names and is found on the shady side of rocks facing north. It is of red, yellow, white, green and black types, among which the red type is superior. It] cures poisoning and chronic fevers.

brag.zhun: **Mineral Exudate:** [a sticky rock exudate] [has eight names and is known in Sanskrit as *shila jatu.* It is found on the north side of rocks and in color is similar to the (red) decoction of dyer's madder. It is of five types, or of six types, according to the more elaborate classification in the Root Tantra. It] is beneficial in all types of fever [and is supreme in curing fevers specifically of the stomach, liver and kidneys. It is also beneficial in wind disorders, especially the 'stiff thigh' wind disorder] and is also unsurpassed as an essence-extraction substance.

(4) Tree Medicines

Tree medicines are [said to be] tenfold: roots, stalks, trunks, branches, petioles, bark, saps, leaves, flowers and fruits. Resins [and secretions] are derived from grasses, trees and animals. Plant medicines are fivefold: roots, stems, leaves, flowers and fruits. [The order of these (ten) is elucidated in the root text as being first, second, third, seventh and eighth. With regard to the sequence from fourth to sixth, some scholars accept that [the series] from camphor to eaglewood includes the tree medicines, and from animal bile to utpala is contained the section on resins. Thence until the beginning of the herb section is contained the plant section. This order is valid. However, in many sections dealing with compounding there are doubts as to the above order] (i.e., the actual classification appears to be contradicted). [In the section of tree medicines (above) there are ten sub-sections, but only four examples are provided.] (N.B. Not all ten parts may be obtained from only four examples), so the three sections, (fourth, fifth and sixth, cannot be expounded in the order of the original ten).

[Here will be explained] the indications and effects of the power [of the individual medicines].

ga.bur: **Camphor:** [has ten names: Bhima tree, *kan(g).tsa, ts(h)ing.ging,* etc. It has a pale yellow trunk, large green leaves, reddish flowers and yellow seeds. There are three types of camphor (resin) namely *shel.ga.bur,* which is white and brittle like ice, *stang.zil,* which is bright yellow with folds, and *mang.ga.bur,* which is in long, bright yellow pieces. All three types] dynamically remove high fevers and totally uproot stubborn chronic fevers.

tsan.dan.dkar.po: **White Sandalwood:** [Red sandal, brown sandal and *su.ru.shug.pa* are a few of the many types of sandalwood. The best type of white sandalwood 'arrow', if placed in boiled butter, will freeze it. It originates from Malaya (the Garlanded Mountain) and there are many varieties. The trunk of the tree is white with green leaves and (distinctive) fragrance.] White sandalwood cures fevers of the lungs and heart and disturbed fever.

tsan.dan.dmar.po: **Red Sandalwood:** [has ten names. It has a red trunk, bright green leaves, red flowers and red, slightly furry, pods. This sandalwood is heavy, resembles horn and has a sweet fragrance. It is of two types, red and brown. It] cures blood fever.

a.ga.ru: **Eaglewood or Aloewood:** *Aquilaria agallocha:* [has eight names. The name *a.ga.ru* means 'not heavy' in Tibetan and the two types are black and yellow. It has bitter taste, coarse power and belongs to the division of warm medicines. The best (black) type has a leaf similar to Artemesia, with green petioles, bright blue flowers and protruding roots, which resemble a wild yak's horn. The yellow type has two sub-types: (the first) has a large trunk, with small, rounded, yellowish-green, furry leaves and fragrant, pale blue flowers; the other yellow type is called *hbah.shig* and has a large brown trunk with bright pale blue flowers. From the grey eaglewood paper is produced, and it has a yellow trunk like a 'meadow cane'. This type has green leaves and bright white flowers.

Eaglewood which boils and gives off a strong smell when placed on the fire is of good quality. It] cures fevers of the heart and life channel.

(5) Resins

gi.wam: **Animal Bile:** [has seven names. The superior type is said to be obtained from the liver of an elephant, but the bile duct of a bull, pig, etc. is also a common source. The brown type is greatly superior to the yellow type]. It cures infectious fever, poisoning, liver fever and vessel organ fever.

chu.gang: **Bamboo Concretion:** [has four names. The real bamboo concretion is found inside the bamboo, and is yellowish-grey with indeterminate taste. The mineral type is white, like salsoda, and is of two types according to quality. Good quality concretion is white and tasteless. It] cures all [types of] lung diseases and removes wound fever.

gur.kum: **Saffron:** *Crocus sativus: Carthamus tinctorius:* [has thirty names. It was brought from 'Fragrant Mountain' by the Arhat Nyi.ma.gung.pa and planted in Kashmir. The best type is reddish-yellow (i.e., the flower) and extremely bright. Nepalese saffron has long stalks as high as a man and large petals, readily visible, with short pistils (which are not obscured by the petals); it is of mediocre quality. Good quality saffron is red and hard. There is little chance of mistaking the saffron which grows in Tibet, and all three types] cure all [types of] liver diseases and constrict the mouths of the channels.

sug.smel: **Smaller Cardamon:** *Elettaria cardamomum:* [has four names. The superior type has a black stalk, green leaf and a white, three-sided pod. *mon.sug* may be used as a substitute for smaller cardamon, which] cures all types of cold kidney [and wind] disorders.

dza.ti: **Nutmeg:** *Myristica fragrans:* [has fifteen names and comes from the *shing.sna.ma* tree. It has a white trunk, green leaves, yellow flowers and malodorous brown fruits which rattle when shaken. It] removes wind disorders and cures heart disorders.

li.shi: **Clove:** [has four names and is of two types. One type resembles a vase whilst the other is similar to a copper nail.] It cures disorders of the life channel, cold wind disorders (and hoarseness).

ka.ko.la: **Greater Cardamon:** *Amomum subulatum:* [has twelve names. It has green leaves and stalk, with thick-skinned, wrinkled fruit. The superior type is hollow and smooth, with thin skin and sharp tips.] It cures cold disorders of the stomach and spleen.

gla.rtsi: **Musk:** [has twenty names. It is obtained from the testicles of the musk deer. The granular type is superior, whilst the inferior type is non-granular.] It cures poisoning, worms, disorders of the kidneys and liver, septic conditions [and infectious disorders (including infectious fevers,) disorders of the eyes and channels, diseases caused by nagas and spirits, and urinary retention].

dom.mkbris: **Bear Bile:** [has seven names. The summer bile is golden whilst the winter bile is turquoise-colored. Good quality bear bile forms a hanging thread in water.] It constricts the mouths of the channels, halts necrosis, grows new flesh [and is beneficial in eye disorders].

ut.pa.la: **Blue Lotus:** *Nelumbo nucifera: Meconopsis:* [has five names. It is of four types depending on the color of the flower, namely, white, red, yellow and blue. The leaves are green and sword shaped with green petioles, and the petioles, buds and leaves are covered with fur. It has seeds similar in size to mustard seeds.] It cures all fevers of the lungs and liver.

na.ga.ge.sar: **Ironwood tree:** *Mesua ferrea: Quisqualis sinensis:* [Three heterogeneous types are found in Nepal and elsewhere. The leaf and trunk resemble the walnut tree and the fruit stalks are thorny. The buds all grow facing in the same direction and the dried red flowers resemble a splayed out copper vessel. It has a white trunk.] *Na.ga pus.pa* [the pistils] cure lung fever, whereas *na.ga ge.sar* [the petals] cure liver fever and *pad.ma ge.sar* [the calyx] cures heart fever.

zi.ra.dkar.po: **(White) Cumin Seed:** *Cuminum cyminum:* [has five names and is a cultivated plant with slender, swordlike, lobed leaves. Its flower is a white umbel and its seed is similar to fennel. The seed has hot and sweet tastes and by its power cures phlegm disorders and indigestion. Yellow cumin (*Bupleurum chinense*) is obtained from the yellow-flowered variety, and both types] cure lung fever.

zi.ra.nag.po: **(Black) Cumin Seed:** *Carum carvi:* [has four names. It has a long, slender, hollow stalk, small blue flowers and small, round, glossy leaves. The seeds are black and three sided, with sweet taste and oily power; they are slightly hot and cure stomach ailments. The Tibetan variety has large leaves and bears the seeds in pods. All claims that it has neither seeds nor flower are unfounded. This type is used to] cure cold disorders of the liver.

la.la.phud: ***Trachyspermum amni* sprague:** *Cnidium monnieri* L.: Skt. *jawani:* [has three names. It has green leaves and stalk and is of three types, according to color: flowers and seeds are white, black or yellow. The seed resembles fennel and the strongest smelling seed indicates the best quality. An inferior type is found in Tibet. All types] cure stomach disorders and cold diseases.

so.ma.ra.dza: **Cannabis medica:** [has thirteen names. It is grown in low lying cultivated areas and has a long, slender trunk. The seed has sweet taste, and is slightly oily (in power) and cures wind disorders, lymph disorders, and worms. The pod is three-sided and contains small, kidney-shaped seeds, and bears the design of a squirrel's (back). The superior type grows in South India and Mon (Nepal, Sikkim and Bhutan) whilst the common type is found everywhere.] It cures skin diseases and lymph conditions.

thal.ka.rdo.rje: **Foetid Cassia:** *Cassia tora:* [has four names. It has small leaves and fruits, slightly bitter taste, and dries lymph (accumulations). It has a green leaf and stem, with yellow flower and yellow wrinkled seed pod. The seed resembles the sex organ of a dog, and the hard type is superior. The common type has a thin seed pod and softer seed, with a band around it. All types] have the same uses as *Cannabis* (above).

gser.gyi.me.tog: **Bitter Cucumber:** *Momordica charantia: Herpetospermum caudigerum* Wall: [has three names. It is a climber with a long thin stem, large leaf and bright yellow flower. The fruit resembles a gimlet.] It cures vessel [organ] fever, bile fever [and the skin is beneficial for hemorrhoids].

gser.gyi.phud.bu: Thladiantha harmsii **Cogn:** [has a fruit similar to a headless *sbur.wa* beetle. It has bitter taste, coarse power, and cures poisoning, phlegm-bile combinations and has an emetic action. This plant is also a creeper with a lined, green petiole and (fruit-) stalk and yellow flower resembling an acorn. The superior type has a bitter, black fruit with coarse power, whilst the common one has a yellow fruit. Both types] act as an emetic in bile disorders.

dug.mo.nyung: **Kurchi:** *Holarrhena antidysenterica* Wall: *Cynanchum sibiricum:* [has twenty names. It has green stalk and leaves and a pale yellow flower. The seed pod is pregnant in appearance and the seed resembles a bird's tongue. The superior type is larger and male, whilst the common type is smaller and female. These] cure bile [disorders] and halt feverish diarrhoea.

144 Quintessence Tantras of Tibetan Medicine

rgun.hbrum: **Raisin:** grape: [has four names. It is a quintessential fruit which grows on forested slopes. The vine has a small round leaf, a tall trunk which resembles the clematis and a small red flower which is difficult to distinguish. The fruit is bright reddish-yellow with sweet, slightly sour taste. Whilst it has the power to halt diarrhoea, excess intake causes diarrhoea. One long-tipped reddish-yellow type of raisin comes from mGo.dkar (in Tibet). From Kashmir is obtained a yellow, seedless raisin, the size of a pea, which is extremely sweet. From Kham come red and black types of raisin, whilst a blue type is obtained from Dag.po. The above types of raisin are in descending order of quality, with the superior type first. They] cure lung disorders and purge fevers.

hu.su: **Coriander:** *Coriandrum sativum:* [has twenty names. Coriander is a superlative medicine. Its leaf, stalk and flower are similar to fennel, whilst the fruit resembles a charm box. Its power removes phlegm disorders and the superior type dispels brown (phlegm). Different types of coriander vary slightly according to the yellowness or blackness of the seeds which] cure stomach phlegm, fever [and thirst, and are beneficial in wind disorders].

star.bu: **Sea Buckthorn:** *Hippophae rhamnoides:* [has fourteen names. It is an extremely coarse, thorny bush with fruit similar to a baby bird. It has a sour taste, pierces the tongue (is very sharp), and cures lung disorders. This plant is also called *ghe.wa.shing,* and is of white and black types. The white type has a small, pea-sized, yellow fruit, which is extremely sour. Prepared in the form of a concentrate] it is expectorant, dissolves blood clots, disperses phlegm, [cures fevers and is beneficial in colic].

bse.yab: **Chaenomeles tibetica:** *Chaenomeles lagenaria:* [The *hKhrungs.dpe* text says, "It is a large tree with a large leaf and a white flower. Its pods contain kernels similar to those of the Bengal Kino tree. It has sour and slightly sweet taste and is of nectarlike benefit in ear diseases. The leaf, trunk and flower resemble the apple tree. One type has a fruit similar to an unripe walnut and does not change color in autumn."] It cures phlegm and fever.

se.hbru: **Pomegranate:** *Punica granatum:* [has seven names and is a hot-natured tree shaped like an umbrella. It has small, round leaves and an extremely attractive white flower. The fruit is shaped like a gourd, is filled with seeds and has sour and sweet tastes with greasy power. It cures cold wind disorders and is supreme in increasing digestive heat.] It cures all stomach disorders, increases digestive heat and removes phlegm and cold disorders.

na.le.sham: **Black Pepper:** *Piper nigrum:* [has four names: *shi.kru, pho.wa.ri, drod.sman* and *ril.mo.* The leaves and trunk are green with thin branches, and the names given above refer to the peppercorns. The white type is called *shi.kru* and both (black and white) types] cure phlegm, cold disorders and erysipelas and are beneficial in nyctalopia.[10]

pi.bi.ling: **Longpeper:** *Piper longum:* [has thirty-three names. The leaf and trunk are green with yellow flowers. The coarse type has elongated seeds of a dull, dark-blue hue and, if classified according to sub-types, the superior or female type is thin and like 'the waist of an ant.' The male type is bulky and both types] cure all cold disorders and wind and spleen disorders.

sman.sga: **Ginger:** *Zingiber officinale:* [has sixteen names. Wild ginger has sweet and hot tastes and heals wounds. Its leaves and petioles are green and the root has a pinkish hue with hard points. Some types appear white and glossy. The different types of ginger, including *don.gra,* increase heat (throughout the body), improve appetite and remove phlegm-wind combinations. Wild ginger includes the sub-type *sgeu.gsher*]. These cure phlegm-wind combinations, dissolve blood clots [and are beneficial for hangovers.]

tsi.tra.ka: **Ceylon Leadwort:** *Plumbago zeylanica:* [has seventeen names. Its taste is extremely hot. The *hKhrungs.dpe* text calls leadwort the king of heat. It grows in hot areas, has flat, undulating leaves and elongated orange pods containing (many) seeds. It has a firelike power to increase (digestive and body) heat, it dispels cold wind disorders and tumors] and cures second-stage oedema, hemorrhoids, worms and leprosy.

shing.tsha: **Cinnamon:** *Cinnamomum tamala:* [has sixteen names and increases (digestive) heat. It grows in thick forest, has a hard trunk, small leaves and both thick and thin types of bark. The thin type is hotter than the thick type, which has balanced power. Cinnamon has hot, sweet, astringent and salty tastes.] It cures cold disorders of the stomach and liver and wind disorders.

karany.ja: **Indian Beech:** *Pongamia pinnata: Caesalpinia sepiaria* Roxb.: [has fourteen names and is said by the Master gYu.thog.pa[11] to be the same as *hjam.hbras* (that is, a different part of the same tree). Others assert it to be *bsrin.bu.dmar.leb* (*mar.ru.tse,* the Bengal Kino tree; Hindi *palasha*). It is the seed of a hot tree, has extremely bitter natural and post-digestive tastes and resembles a snake's egg. Indian beech is of black and green types and is very rare nowadays.] It increases digestive heat.

shing.kun: **Asafoetida:** *Ferula narthex:* [has fourteen names and is of two types. One is the resin of the Pokka tree. A white thread rubbed against this tree will turn blue. The other type is radishlike and the root is half exposed above the ground. It is pale yellow and contains a milky sap.] It is a vermifuge and cures cold disorders and heart wind.

byi.tang.ga: ***Embelia ribes:*** [has four names. It has a long, thin trunk, small, pale, coarse leaves with small reddish-blue flowers, and fruits like chickpeas scattered by hailstones. (The fruit) has sweet and sour tastes and] cures worm and parasitic infestations and increases digestive heat.

ma.ru.tse: **Bengal Kino Tree:** *Butea frondosa:* [has eight names and grows in hot areas. It has a blue, coarse leaf and slender trunk, a yellow flower and orange fruit. It has bitter and sweet tastes, is an anthelmintic and] cures phlegm and rheumatism.

go.bye: ***Semecarpus anacardium:*** *Momordica cochinchinensis:* [is of black and white types. The skin of the fruit is drawn together like the mouth of a bag and its juice resembles blood.] It is a vermifuge, removes bone-[growths] and cures stomach infections.

spos.dkar: **Resin of White Saltree:** *Shorea robusta: Boswellia:* [has seven names, for example, *gu.gul.dkar.po,* etc. It has a brown trunk with bright yellow hue, green leaves, a yellow flower and white resin the color of horses' teeth.] It purges lymph [accumulations] and dries them at their [respective] location. [The common black type has no medicinal application.]

gu.gul: **Indian Bedellium Tree:** *Commiphora mukul:* [has eleven names and is also known as *(shing.)hdre.hjigs.* It is of two types: white and black. The trunk is reddish-yellow, with many layers of bark and green leaves. The clear, dark resin of this tree constitutes the white type, whilst the black type is dark and opaque. Both types dispel [nagas, infectious diseases caused by spirits], earth spirits, infectious tissue degeneration, [anterior transposition of the calf muscle], painful infectious disorders, [wind disorders and 'the stiff thigh' wind disorder].

shel.ta: **Pine Resin:** *Pinus griffithii:* [has three names: *thang.chu,* etc.] It retains bone resin and bone lymph.

rgya.tsha: **Lake Salt:** [has seven names. It resembles calcite, and has a hot taste similar to *mtshur* (alunite).] It is a vermifuge, neutralizes [all types of] poisons, purges channel disorders, removes quinsy and diphtheria, removes waste-growths of the flesh, and cures urinary retention.

rgyam.tsha: **Rock Salt:** [has nine names and is a clear, crystalline salt obtained from stone. It resembles male calcite *(pho.chong)* and has slightly sweet taste.] Rock salt cures phlegm-wind combinations, indigestion and cold disorders.

lche.myang.tsha: **Wood Salt:** [is (derived from) the branch of a tree, grows in hot areas, for example southern valleys, and has a reddish hue. This and rock salt are the superior types of salt]. Wood salt is also [applied in the] same [way as rock salt and] is beneficial for the eyes.

kha.ru.tsha: **Black 'Sanchal' Salt:** [has nine names and is of red and black types. That of superior quality is very clear, whilst artificial black salt is common.]

tsabs.ru.tsha: **White Mineral Salt:** Crag halite: [has five names and is of natural and artificial types. Good quality white mineral salt is white and resembles *mdung.rtse,* whilst the artificial type is a white salt]. Both black and white mineral salt increase [digestive] heat, treat distention [of the abdomen], belching, flatulence and phlegm-wind combinations.

rwa.tsha and *thal.tsha:* **Horn Salt** and **Ash Salt:** [are both artificial salts of no fixed color and] cure cold disorders of the vessel organs.

mdze.tsha: **White Rock Salt:** [resembles clear, dried bubbles of *mtshur* (alunite) on rocks]. It dissolves blood clots and drains [accumulations of] lymph from wounds.

tsha.la: **Borax:** [has five names, *dar.tshur, dar.sman,* etc. It originates from lakes and the superior type is crystalline in

appearance. The common type is called *bye.brun.ma* and both
types] heal wounds, dissolve blood clots, act as a purgative [and
dry lymph accumulations].

lba.tsha: **Soda Salt:** Saltpetre: [is a type of salt which resembles crystalline lumps of 'rock sugar.' It has an extremely strong,
salty taste and] dispels goiters. [Moreover when soda salt is not
available the salt from cave floors is a suitable substitute].

a.ru.ra: **Chebulic Myrobalan:** *Terminalia chebula:* [has
eleven names. The *hKrungs.dpe* text states, "Chebulic myrobalan
has a large trunk, thick green leaves and a yellow flower. The
number of the different types of fruit is said to be eight, seven
or five. The bark resembles that of a walnut tree and the middle
bark is greenish-yellow. The fruits may be black or yellow with
eight or five sub-types of the yellow one."] Chebulic myrobalan
has five tastes, excluding saltiness, is life-giving, increases
[digestive] heat, acts as a digestive and is wholesome [for the
body]. It cures all diseases arising from wind, bile and phlegm.
The five types are *rnam.rgyal* ('victor'), *hjigs.med* ('fearless'),
bdud.rtsi ('nectar'), *hphel.byed* ('increasing'), and *skem.po*
('dry').

rnam.par.rgyal.wa ('victor') has six names. It was only
available in the time of gYu.thog.pa.[11] It resembles the 'neck'
of a gourd [and has all six tastes]. However, the fruit of the
gser.mdog type has a 'neck' and is larger [than that of any other
type]. It is a suitable substitute but if one could obtain the actual
'Victor' type the advantages would be that it cures disorders of
the three humors, wind, bile and phlegm, a well as all hot and
cold disorders. The presence of this fruit is particularly auspicious
and favorable [like a wish-fulfilling gem] in fulfilling all aims.

hjigs.med ('fearless') [has six names] and five facets. [It is
black, extremely elongated] and is recommended in eye
diseases and against [different types of] spirits.

bdud.rtsi ('nectar') [has six names and is also known as
Sham.Thug. The fruit is yellow and has thick flesh.] It enables
one to gain weight.

hphel.byed ('increasing') [has three names and] is rounded
like a vase. It is recommended for wounds.

skem.po ('dry') [has two names. The fruit has thin flesh and]
many folds. It cures bile disorders in children.

[Other types include *gser.mdog,* which is yellow; the long-tipped variety known as *mchu.snyung* or *haritaka* in Sanskrit; and *nag.chung*, which has no kernel.]

ba.ru.ra: **Beleric Myrobalan:** *Terminalia belerica:* [has eleven names. It is a large tree with a pale yellow trunk, dull, flat leaves and small white flowers. The fruit is smoother than that of chebulic myrobalan and the good quality type is small and yellow. The common type has a larger fruit. Both varieties] cure phlegm and bile disorders, lymph disorders [and wind imbalances].

skyu.ru.ra: **Emblic Myrobalan:** *Emblica officinalis:* [has eleven names. It grows in hot areas and has a tall, supple trunk with large leaves and dull, orange flowers. The whitish fruit is of good quality, whilst the black one is common. Both types] cure phlegm and bile disorders, blood diseases, [wind imbalances and polyuria].

snying.zho.sha: Spondias axillaris **Roxb.:** [has two names. *hKhrungs.dpe* text says, "It is the type of Spondias that cures heart diseases and grows in forested valleys. (The tree) has a large trunk and thick leaves. The flower is white and extremely attractive, whilst the fruit is heart-shaped, black and coarse]. It cures heart fevers."

mkhal.zho.sha: **Cowhage:** *Canavalia gladiata: Mucuna prurita:* [*hKhrungs.dpe* says, "Cowhage has a slender trunk and smooth leaves. The flower is attractive and indigo-hued whilst the yellow pods contain black kidney-shaped seeds of sweet taste and oily power. These seeds cure kidney disorders and the white type is superior to the black or yellow types]. It cures kidney fever."

gla.gor.zho.sha: **Entada scandens:** *Entada phaseoloides:* [is also known as *mchher.pa.zho.sha* or *glang.mig* (lit. 'spleen power or bulls eye') and is likely to be mistaken for cowhage. It has a small, slender trunk, thick round leaf and white flower. The heart-shaped pods contain black and white striped kidney-shaped seeds which are thick at the center. The spleen-shaped one is of superior quality and] cures spleen fever.

a.hbras: **Mango Kernel:** *Mangifera indica: Terreya nucifera:* [has four names. The tree has a small trunk with a leaf similar to that of Himalayan rhubarb. It has blue umbrella-shaped flowers and sweet and sour fruit resembling a stag's testicle.]

sra.hbras: **Schizandra chinensis:** *Milletia pachycarpa:*

Eugenia jambolana: Smilax bockii: [has two names. It is a tree of moderate size with leaves similar to *spa.ma* (a type of juniper). The seeds are small, black, hard and vase-shaped.]

hjam.hbras: **Indian Beech:** *Pongamia pinnata: Pongamia glabra: Caesalpinia crista:* [is said to be the same as *karany.ja* and has seven names. It has a large black trunk, scattered thorny leaves, yellow flower and a long pod, containing green seeds which rattle. This, (mango kernel and *Schizandra chinensis*)] cure (cold) kidney disorders.

hbra.go: **Date:** *Polygonum convulvulus:* [has sweet taste. The trunk is red with green leaves and yellow, white or blue flowers. The fruit of the supreme type is known as *a.mrar.* One type has a red, thorny trunk with green leaves, white flowers and a fruit which resembles a horse's teat. It is also known as *ha.re.nu.ka, ma.nu.rta.ska* or *chhi.pa.khar.* It] cures brown and yellow phlegm and stomach disorders [and in addition is beneficial in wind fever, blood fever, insanity caused by spirits and as an aphrodisiac].

ma.nu.pa.tra: **Iris germanica Linn:** *Aristolochia* sp.: *Inula racemosa:* [has five names. The leaves are turquoise-coloured with silver, furry backs and grow upwards. The root is white and flowers are bright yellow and well-scented. It has hot and bitter tastes, with sweet and sour post-digestive tastes]. It cures wind and blood disorders and fevers.

pushkaramula: **Inula racemosa:** *Aplotaxis lappa: Iris germanica: Vladimiria souliei:* [has five names and is said to be the root of *Iris germanica,* etc. It is cultivated and has a flower and leaf similar to dock-leaf. The root is white and] cures phlegm fevers.

ru.rta: **Costus Root:** *Saussurea lappa: Costus speciosus:* [has ten names. It has yellowish-green leaf, white flower and black or white antler-like roots] It dispels wind and blood disorders, abdominal distension, lung diseases, diphtheria, quinsy, throat abscesses, etc., and [superfluous] flesh growths. [Costus root is identified in many different ways, and the scholars of antiquity classified eight different types. Even (the type of *ma.nu* known as) *ma.nu.shu.zur (Iris germanica)* has been variously identified, for example, as having green leaves, white flowers and yellow bark on the stalks and petioles. One type of *ma.nu* called *se.shing* is a climber on trees such as bamboo or cedar pine, and has pale leaves. Other types of *ma.nu* may be studied in their respective chapter as they are of less importance in the present section.]

yung.wa: **Turmeric:** *Curcuma longa:* [has three names. The leaf is similar to that of garlic. The root bark is reddish-yellow and (in Tibet) it is known as yellow ginger. It has slightly bitter taste and] neutralizes poison, halts necrosis, dispels infectious diseases (and is beneficial in polyuria).

shu.dag: **Sweet Flag (root):** *Acorus calamus:* [has seven names. It grows in water and the leaves resemble rice shoots. The root is of black and white types and has hot taste and coarse power. The white root is fragrant and sweet tasting, is used in naga medicines and wisdom pills and is beneficial in poisoning. The black root is more commonly recommended in medicine and both types] cure indigestion, increase digestive heat, and cure throat abcesses, [all types of infectious disorders], [disease caused by] spirits and lymph disorders.

pu.shel: **Khus-khus Grass:** *Vetiveria zizanioides: Dendrobium curcuminatum: Belamacanda chinensis:* [has eleven names. It grows on river banks, has stalks similar to kusha grass, and the root smells like camphor]. It halts vomiting, cures phlegm fever [and hemorrhoids, and relieves urinary retention].

White and brown hkhyung.sder (lit. 'garuda's talon'): ***Uncaria rhynchophylla:*** *Nauclea rhynchophylla:* [The white type resembles a garuda's talon, whilst the brown type is similar to a crow's foot. The former type has black petioles and green leaf. Both types] cure [all kinds of] fever [caused by] poisoning.

dpah.wo: ***Phytolacca esculenta*** (white type): ***Scutellaria baicalensis:*** *Phytolacca acinosa* (yellow type): [For example, the yellow type grows in soft ground, has small yellow flower and a hollow yellow root. It has bitter taste, cool power and neutralizes poison. This yellow type is distinct only by virtue of its color and is beneficial in horse and mule diseases. The wild type resembles the white one (but has roots shaped like potatoes with tendrils), and is known as *nar.ma.nur.mar.* All three types] cure fever caused by poisoning.

bong.nga.dkar.po: **White Aconite:** *Aconitum naviculare* Stapf.: *Aconitum sinense: Aconitum heterophyllum:* [has ten names and is of four types: white, red, yellow and black. The black type is highly toxic, whilst the white one has bitter taste and neutralizes poison. The latter has small, pointed leaves with seven or eight lobes. The stalk is small and supple, and the flowers are pale blue with a reddish hue]. It cures infectious fever with poisoning and bile fever.

bong.nga.dmar.po: **Red Aconite:** *Aconitum* sp.: [has a crimson flower and a red root. It has bitter taste and is an antidote to poison].

bong.nga.ser.po: **Yellow Aconite:** *Aconitum autumnale:* [has a yellowish flower. It has bitter taste, cool power and is recommended in poison fevers and infectious bile fever. (Roots of) red and yellow aconite] cure meat poisoning and poisoning from black aconite (*Aconitum ferrox* Wall).

shing.mngar: **Liquorice:** *Glycyrrhiza glabra:* [has fifteen names. It has yellowish-green sessile leaves. The superior or male type is cultivated, whilst the female species grows near river banks, and the neuter type grows in forested areas near river banks. It has a yellow root, a sweet taste and] cures lung diseases and channel disorders.

sle.tres: **Heart-leaved Moonseed:** *Tinospora cordifolia:* [has seven names. It has sweet taste, cures various diseases and is a primary ingredient in essence-extraction compounds. Moonseed is a yellowish-blue climber containing many small (white) glands, and is beneficial in gout.]

kanda.ka.ri: **Indian Salamin:** *Solanum xanthocarpum: Rubus saxatilis:* [has twenty names. Its woody stem resembles that of the young wild rose and it has a bright pale yellow flower. Salamin (is a small thorny herb) bearing clusters of red berries having sweet and astringent tastes]. Moonseed and salamin cure wind fevers, [infectious fevers and cough].

ga.dra: **Brown Salamin:** *Rubus idaeus: Debregeasia edulis: Solanum indicum:* [has fourteen names, for example *stag.tsher (Salsola collina)* and *brihati*]. It too is beneficial [in wind fever and] infectious fever.

tig.ta: **Chiretta:** *Swertia chirata:* [has six names. One type known as *rgya.tig* has dark blue or yellowish-green petioles, the interior of which is soft. The leaves grow in opposite pairs at intervals along the stalk. This species with its blossoming yellow flower is the superior type. There is also a Nepalese type and a common type from Tibet. All three types] cure all types of bile fever.

ba.sha.ka: **Malabar Nut Tree:** *Adhatoda vasica: Veronica ciliata Fisch:* [has twelve names. It grows in forested south-facing valleys, has a large trunk, thick leaves and bright pale yellow flowers, with bitter taste and cool power. Of the many types the white, red and blue ones are superior and a mediocre type is found in Tibet]. It cures blood fevers, [poisoning, painful infectious fevers, liver diseases and bile disorders].

*ba.le.ka: **Aristolochia saccata** Wall* (a type of birthwort): *Aristolochia contorta: Akebia quinata: Menispermum dahuricum:* [has six names and is a twining shrub similar to clematis which has no fruit nor flower. It has bitter taste, coarse power and cures phlegm, painful infectious fever and blood disorders]. Birthwort also cures fevers of the lungs, liver and vessel organs.

(li.)ga.dur: **Meadow Cranesbill:** *Geranium pratense: Erodium stephanium: Bergenia crassifolia: Rhodiola wallichiana:* [The male type has seven names and the female type has six. It has balanced hot and cold power, hot and sweet tastes, cures lung disorders and reduces swellings. It has thick leaves similar to rice shoots, and the root resembles a withered gland. The flower has a pink interior and resembles a bird's beak. The common variety grows in Tibet and has pink petioles. All types] cure infectious fevers, lung fevers and channel fevers.

*stab.seng: **Eucommia ulmoides:** Fraxinus rhynchophylla:* [has five names and is said to be a white or blue type of the *spyi.zhur* tree (*Terminalia tomentosa*). It grows in forested, south-facing valleys and has bark similar to that of *shyar.pa* (poplar). The leaf is pale green, and a fragment of the middle bark placed in water leaves a pillar-like trace]. It unites fractures and cures bone fevers.

sgron.shing: **Yew-leaf Fir:** *Pinus picea: Pinus massionana: Pinus tabulaeformis: Pinus silvestris:* [has three names, for example *rasna*, etc. It has hot taste and dry, coarse power. It has a large trunk, scattered needles, a long, scented cone and yields a resinous oil upon combustion]. It cures wind-phlegm combinations, cold lymph disorders [and dispels tumors. The root is beneficial in gynecological disorders].

skyer.pa: **Indian Barberry:** *Berberis aristata: Berberis* *asiatica:* [has eleven names and cures poisoning, chronic infectious fevers and eye disorders. It has silvery bark, a yellow flower and a red (or blue) berry.] The [yellow] middle bark cures bile disorders and kidney fevers and is beneficial for the eyes.

se.rgod: **Wild Rose:** *Rosa avicularis: Rosa sericea: Rosa laevigate:* [has two names. With respect to the female type, the interior of the stem is red with brown bark and red flower. The roots resemble iron hooks and the hips are reddish-green and furry. The stem of the male type is hollow, brown and without thorns]. Indian barberry and wild rose collect toxins and cure lymph disorders. [Wild rose is also recommended for use in disorders caused by spirits.]

seng.ldeng: **Catechu Tree:** *Acacia catechu:* [has twenty-three names, and the trunk is large and extremely hard. The leaves resemble pig's bristles, and its taste is slightly bitter. Different types of catechu according to color include *tsan.dan.seng.ldeng* (lit. 'sandal catechu'), *skyer.seng.ldeng* (lit. 'barberry catechu') and *gsom.seng.ldeng*. The concentrate of catechu is known as *khyi.la.wa.ri*]. It dries (bad) blood and lymph accumulations.

so.cha: **Soapnut Tree:** *Sesbania grandiflora: Randia dumetorum: Aesculus chinensis:* [has nine names. It has hot taste, slightly oily power and is an emetic in all types of phlegm disorders. The trunk is large, white and hard with thin glossy leaves and pale yellow flowers. The nut resembles an old man's testicle and contains a kernel similar to the castor oil seed, the castor bean]. It is the supreme all-round emetic for all diseases.

dan.rog: **Castor Oil Plant:** *Croton tiglium:* [has seven names and is an emetic and purgative of phlegm and tri-humoral disorders. It has a green trunk and leaf, though sometimes these may be red. The trunk and petioles are hollow, and the leaves may have nine or five pointed lobes. It has white flowers and thorny pods containing extremely soft, black beans known as *dza.yi.pha.la*. The latter is considered to be the superior type.]

dan.khra: ***Ricinus communis:*** [grows in shady forested places as a climber on tall trees. It has a slightly coarse leaf and striped kernel similar to the above type, and also resembles the seed of *sbur.wa.ske.bchad*. The inferior type has a black kernel resembling a frog's back].

shri.khanda: ***Euphorbia*** sp.: *Fritillaria verticillata: Stewartia* sp.: [has eight names. *'shri.khanda'* means *dpal.gyi.dum.bu* (lit. 'a fragment of the Lord'). It is a large, blue tree with spreading branches not unlike an old man. It has astringent and slightly bitter tastes, and the branches yield a white, curdlike sap which is melted to make the concentrate. The inferior type grows in Nepal and elsewhere, and is a rounded, leafless plant containing similar sap]. Castor oil seed and *shri.khanda* are drastic purgatives. [The latter also heals abscesses].

dong.ga: **(Purging) Cassia:** Cassia pods: *Cassia fistula* Linn: [has seven names: It has sweet and slightly hot taste and purges all types of disease. Purging cassia is a climber which grows in hot areas and has large leaves. The pod resembles an intestine filled with blood]. It cures liver disorders and is a mild laxative.

ka.ped: a type of **Bael Fruit:** *Aegle marmelos* Corr: *Citrullus vulgaris: Cucurbita pepo: Lagenaria siceraria:* [has thirteen names. It has slightly sour taste and heals wounds and lung diseases. *ka.ped* is a climber similar to bitter cucumber. The leaves are similar to those of *ha.lo* (hollyhock) in bloom. *ka.ped* is the male type and takes the form of a light red gourd carried by sadhus as a water vessel. The female type is called *bilwa*.]

da.trig: **Schizandra:** *Schizandra sphaerandra* Stapf. f. *pallida* Smith: *Rhus semilata:* [has seven names. It has sweet and sour tastes and grows in hot areas. The trunk is large and hard with grey bark, a small red flower and berries which resemble the eggs of sheep's lice.]

smag: **Powdered Root** of, for example, old pine trees: *Padus asiatica:* [has three names and is of red and white types].

mon.chha.ra: **Indian Oak (Acorn):** *Quercus semicarpifolia* Sm: *Quercus lanuginosa: Quercus acutissima:* [has six names. It has a rounded tea plant-like leaf, small thorns and fruits similar to nutmeg. The black type yields a blood(-like resin)].
Aegle marmelos, Schizandra, pine root and acorn halt all types of hot and cold diarrhoea.

(7) Exposition of the Powers of Herbs[12]
hong.len: **Picrorhiza:** *Picrorhiza Kurroa: Picrorhiza scrofulariaefolia: Lagotis glauca:* [has seven names, *pu.tse.shel,* etc. It grows in rocky meadows, has blue flowers resembling vultures' droppings, furry fierce-bladed leaves and a root similar to an earthworm. The inferior species is of male and

female types, of which the latter is non-flowering]. Picrorhiza
dries [bad] blood, cures disturbed fever, vital organ fever [and
wind disorders, for example, 'stiff thigh' (*brla.rengs*)].

spang.rtsi.do.wo: **Pterocephalus hookeri Hook:** *Saussurea
nepalensis:* [has ten names and includes three types of
chig.thub.dkar.po used in infectious fevers of the small intestine.[13] It has large, plain leaves, bitter taste, a white flower
similar to the head of an old man and long petioles. The sub-
species cures disturbed infectious fever.]

[The second type,] *(shrang.rtsi.)hbyar.bag.(chan),* [is similar and cures urinary disorders, polyuria, chronic diseases and
fever of the urinary bladder.]

lug.rtsi: **Saussurea uniflora:** [has dark fragrant flowers. All
three types] cure infectious fever, poisoning and chronic fevers.

re.skon: **Corydalis edulis:** *Potentilla tanacetifolia: Potentilla
supina:* [has seven names, for example, *rtsi.dmar* and *phug.ron.
rkang.bchas.* It grows in rocky meadows, has spreading leaves
like *Nelumbium nucifer* ('utpala') and a single root with eight
tendrils. The flower is yellow and retains dewdrops. It is well-
scented and has extremely bitter taste]. Corydalis is hemostatic
and cures channel fever caused by brown phlegm [and
dysentery with fever].

kyi.lche: **Gentiana straminea** Maxim: *Swertia petiolata*
(white type): [has fourteen names, for example, *sha.lang,* etc.
It has long, smooth, thick green leaves and white flowers
similar to *Gentiana algida (spang.rgyan).* The stalk is red, and
the seeds are so dark as to resemble iron filings. The taste is
bitter with coarse power. The black type (*Gentiana dahurica*)
grows in shady places and has thinner leaves than the white
type. It has a blue-brown flower and petiole, reduces swellings
and cures scrofula.[14] Both types] cure vessel organ fever and
bile fever.

sum.chu.tig: **Saxifraga pasumensis** Marq. et Shaw. f.
integrifolia Jesir: *Gentiana amarella:* [grows in rocky meadows and has small, flat green leaves like the beak of the *rko.ma*
bird. It has clusters of small, pale yellow flowers similar to
lotuses and reddish-yellow furry stems]. It cures liver fever and
bile fever.

pri.yang.ku: **Callicarpa macrophylla** Vahl or
Dracocephalum tangutium Maxim: [has six names, *rtsi.hu,* etc.

It has bitter-sweet taste, is hemostatic, heals wounds, dries
lymph accumulations, cures all types of liver fevers and has
inconceivable qualities. The petioles are thin, with blue leaves
and flowers]. It cures fevers of the stomach and the liver.

zangs.tig: **Gentiana** sp.: *Gueldenstaedtia multiflora* (a type
of red gentian): [grows in dry places, has a green leaf and petals
a little like those of the mustard flower. It has red petioles, many
branching stems, a pale red flower and bitter taste.] Red gentian
cures infectious fevers.

lchags.tig: **Gentianopsis paludosa** (Monro) Ma:
Lomatogonium sp.: [has two names and grows in clumps. It has
small leaves, (long) blue flowers (with pointed petals) and thin,
black petioles. Its taste is bitter and it cures wound fevers and
infectious fevers]. Both red gentian and Gentianopsis cure bile
fevers.

gser.tig: **Swertia angustifolia:** *Swertia wolfgangiara:*
Swertia vacillans: [has a yellowish-green leaf (like) the beak of
the *rko.ma* bird and bluish-yellow flowers spotted like the
ngur.pa bird. It has bitter taste and cures disorders of blood,
bile and infectious fevers].

sro.lo: **Rhodiola saera** (Prain) Fu: *Strobilanthes japonicus*
(red type):

sug.hdra: **Solms-Laubachia eurycarpa** (Maxim) Botsch.:
Gypsophila dahurica (brown type): [*sro.lo* is of two types. The
white one (*Cochlearia scapiflora: Cochlearia rusticana:
Platycodon grandiflorum*) grows in rocky, snowy mountains
and has a thin root with large trunk and bark. It has a thick,
glossy leaf and an extremely attractive white flower. White
sro.lo cures lung diseases and dysentery]. *sug.hdra,* [the brown
type, has a single-stranded root whence springs the trunk,
brown petioles, white flower bearing dewdrops and large, flat,
crescent moon-shaped pod. There is also a subspecies of this
type with thin pods. (All types of *sro.lo*)] cure lung fevers.

gyah.kyi.ma: **Pyrola incarnata:** *Pyrola rotundifolia:*
Chrysoplenium nepalense: [is also known as *zla.wa.bsil.
wahi.bdud.rtsi* (lit. 'cool moon nectar') and grows on cliffs. It
has a pale blue leaf and flower, bitter taste and is an all-round
emetic. The large-flowering variety is the king type, and the
small-flowering one is the queen type. It is also classified
according to yellow, white, red and blue or gold, silver, copper

and iron types]. *Pyrola* pacifies and purges [all types of] bile disorders.

gang.ga.chhung: **Gentiana urnula** H.sim: *Gentiana depressa: Leonurus sibiricus:* [grows in rocky meadows and is a four-pointed, eight-sided, banner-shaped plant with a bell-shaped flower. It has bitter taste and cool power and] dispels poisoning and dysentery caused by fever.

bya.rgod.spos: **Delphinium brunonianum** Royle: *Delphinium cashmirianum:* [has six names. It grows in rocky meadows, has thick leaves and a pale blue, musk scented, furry flower shaped like an owl's head]. It dispels spirits, infectious fever with poisoning and heals insect bites.

yu.mo.srol.gong.wa: a type of **Soroseris hookeriana** Stebb: *Lactuca sibirica:* [grows in rocky meadows and has bluish-green leaves similar to those of dandelion. It has a hollow, bulky, comb-shaped flower of blue, yellow or white type. The root is extremely bitter and] heals skull fractures and fever with poisoning.

yu.mo.mde.hbyin: **Paraquilegia microphylla** Royle: *Dianthus superbus: Erodium stephanium:* [grows on rocks, etc., and has scattered bluish-green leaves. It is of white, red and blue flowering types with yellow pistils and] induces expulsion of a dead fetus and acts as a painkiller by ejecting [bullets, etc., lodged in the body].

dar.ya.kan[15]: **Moerhingia latifolia** (L) Tenzl.: *Draba nemorosa: Scabiosa comosa: Lepidium apetalum: Lepidium latifolium: Astragalus tongolensis* Ulbr.: [is a rare and secret medicine with boundless qualities and has been classified in various ways by different scholars. It grows between rocks and has a thin three-pointed leaf. It has a bitter yellow root and, when compounded, cures the four hundred and four kinds of disease. The leaf and root vary from pale blue, whilst the flowers may be bluish and slightly brown or pale yellow, blue or red. It has long thin pods containing small black seeds and stiff leaves and trunk. The white-flowered type has four petals, and its seed resembles lapis. In the *Kalacakra Tantra* it is known as *kha.rag.krod. dar.ya.kan* has green leaf and petiole and] dries lymph accumulations in the chest, unites skull fractures, maintains bone resin [and is beneficial in oedema].

rta.lpags (lit. 'horse skin'): a type of **Lamiophlomis rotata**

(Benth) Kude: *Marrubium incisum: Colqhounia coccinea:* [is of hills- and plains-growing types and has thick, round speckled leaves and a thorny, four-sided stalk. The flower may be pink or white. The hill variety has bitter-sweet taste and treats worm infestations, whilst the plains variety has warm, dry power]. It maintains bone resin and drains lymph accumulations.

a.bi.sha or *a.bi.ka* (lit. 'non-poison'): **Fritillaria delavayi** Franch.: *Fritillaria cirrhosa: Lilium nepalense: Uraria crinita:* [has six names. It has a brown hanging flower, brown trunk, green petiole and six-sided pod containing flat seeds. Fritillaria has sweet taste, cool power and] heals skull fractures and fever caused by poisoning.

stag.sha (lit. 'tiger flesh'): **Potentilla discolor:** *Calophaca crassicaulis: Oxytropis chiliophylla* Royle (white type): [has five names. It has slightly bitter taste and subdues spirits by its sweet fragrance. The white variety has a green leaf and stalk and a single root from which many stalks branch out. The flower is reddish-blue, slightly coarse and is in the form of three-sided ears (cff. corn). The black or blue type has a yellowish-green leaf, smaller than the white type, as well as a large pod. It has a strong odor]. It heals wounds, cures septic disorders and poisoning, [halts dysentery, reduces swellings and acts as an emetic].

spang.rgyan.dkar.po: **Gentiana algida** Pall (white type): *Gentiana triflora:* [has a bitter taste, small elongated green leaves and a white, blue or striped flower]. It cures throat disorders, fever caused by poisoning [and infectious fever].

yu.gu.shing: **Veronica longiflora:** *Veronica incana: Senecio dianthus* Franch (white type): *Cacalia quinquelobus: Sambucus adnata* Wall (black type of elder): [has nine names. The brown type is said to be *dar.ya.kan,* and it grows in very hot areas. The white type has a large lobed leaf, pale green on top and brown beneath. It has small, slightly furry flowers, bitter taste, cool power and subdues spirits by its pungent odor. The plains-growing black type has dandelion-like dark green leaves. Both types] heal wounds, cure fever caused by poisoning [and dispel spirits].

rtsad: **Pleurospermum** species of *rtsad.rgod* (wild type): *Pleurospermum hookeri* C.B. Clarke: [has two names. It has a black petiole, flat, greenish-brown, hollow seed, fine, smooth, blue leaf, erect stalk and pale yellow flower. No toxic plants ever grow in the vicinity of this herb. The common type grows on hard ground, has a lobed leaf, thin stalk and small white flower similar to that of fennel. It has bitter taste, coarse power and cures all types of fever].

rgu.thub or glang.chen.chig.thub: **Scutellaria baicalensis:** [grows on shady, rocky hills and has a large 'elephant-like' root. It has small leaves and flowers and dark red umbrella-like fruit. The common type is the yellow type of *dpah.wo (Scutellaria)* with leaf and petiole, known as *glang.chen,* and has a huge tap-root. It has bitter and astringent tastes, cool power and] cures all types of fevers.

ldum.stag: **Strychnos nux-vomica:** [has five names, for example, *rgya.mtso.ldum.stsag, go.byi.la,* etc., and grows in hot areas as a climber on large trees. It has a white blue-tinged stalk, green leaf, white flower and yellow pod. *Strychnos* has a bitter taste and coarse power, and its seed is called *bya.hphur.leb*).

Pleurospermum, Scutellaria and *Strychnos* cure poisoning.

a.byag: **Chrysanthemum tatsiense:** *Inula britannica: Tanacetum* sp.: *Pyrethrum barbigera:* [is also known as *gzer.hjoms* and has five names. It has slightly bitter taste and cures infectious tissue degeneration. The stalk is flexible with a yellow flower like a golden umbrella and a dark green coarse leaf]. It heals skull fractures, dries lymph accumulations [and is beneficial in painful infectious fever].

tsher.sngon: **Blue Poppy:** *Meconopsis horridula* Hook f. et Thoms: [has four names and grows on high, rocky hills and mountains. It has a small sword-like green leaf, brown petiole, attractive blue flower with yellow stamens and is rendered very coarse by a covering of fine thorns. Blue poppy has a bitter taste and] heals skull fractures, sustains bone resin [and cures bone fever].

smug.chhung.mdan.yon: a type of **Blue Poppy:** *Meconopsis integrifolia:* [is called by some *smug.chhung.ber.mgo* and has a green sword-shaped leaf. It has a brown flower with yellow stamens and resembles blue poppy in being covered with fine thorns, whilst its taste is slightly bitter]. It has the same uses [as blue poppy].

gser.skud (lit. 'gold thread'): **Cuscuta sinensis:** *Usnea* *diffracta: Parmelia saxatilis:* [has a slender yellow stalk and bitter taste. The white stalked type is bulkier and is known as *dngul.skud* ('silver thread'). It has bitter taste and] cures fevers of the lungs, liver and channels, and also fever caused by poisoning.

*lug.ru (smug.po):***Pedicularis oliveriana** Prain: *Pedicularis pectinata: Pedicularis pyramidate:* [is also known as *thal.tre* and is of red, yellow and brown types. It has a long, lobed green leaf and a brown flower bearing the design of a sheep's horn. Brown *Pedicularis* has bitter taste, fluid power and] collects poisons, cures meat poisoning, [brown phlegm, channel fever, dysentery with fever, stimulates hair growth and turns grey hair black. Red *Pedicularis* differs from the above by the color of the flower.]

lug.ru.ser.po: **Pedicularis longiflora** Rudolph var. *tubiformis* (Klotz) Tsoong: *Pedicularis tenuirostris: Pedicularis bicomuta:* [grows in shady meadows and has a yellow flower similar to that of the brown type. It collects poisons and dries 'reservoirs' of pus.]

chhu.rug (sbal.lag): **Halerpestes sarmentosa** (Adams): [has four names and grows near rivers, even during winter. It has a turquoise root similar to a coiled snake and a turquoise leaf shaped like frogs' feet. The inferior type has a heavily lobed leaf. Both types, as well as] *Pedicularis* (above) dry fluid accumulations [and *Halerpestes sarmentosa* cures bone fever].

Se.wahi.me.tog: **Wild Rose:** *Rosa roxburghii: Rosa sericea* Lindl: *Rosa avicularis:* [has five names and is of black and white types. It is a large thorny bush with small, round, slightly coarse leaves, white flower and red hips. It has sweet and sour tastes, and oily power, and] cures bile disorders and alleviates wind imbalances.

hbu.su.hang: **Lotus corniculata:** *Medicago sativa: Trigonella pubescens:* [has three names and grows in fields. It has a glossy seed pod and cures fevers of the kidneys, lungs and heart. The female type has a rough leaf and stalk, and yellow flowers and seed pods. The male type has slender spreading petioles, small round green leaves, yellow flowers and is without pods. Both types] heal wounds and cure lung diseases.

sgong.thog.pa or *sgong.thog.hbar:* **Erysimum altaicum:** *Erysimum diffusum* Ehrh.: [has five names. It has a white taproot, a leaf and petiole similar to the mustard plant, single stalk, yellow flower and thin seed pod containing yellow seeds known as *hdre.pad.kha*]. It cures meat poisoning, disturbed fever, [lung diseases, blood disorders and smallpox].

a.krong (white type): **Arenaria capillaris** Poir: *Stellaria palustris* Ehrh. (common type): *Gypsophila dahurica: Artemesia spice: Artemesia hedinii* (black type): [is of four types, i.e., *mkhan.pa.a.krong, phur.mo.a.krong* and two types of *rtsa.a.krong* explained below which are glossy with dewdrops. The black type has a small stalk, thin petioles and blue scattered leaves with small indentations. The white type has a thick leafstalk, large leaves and yellow flowers. The tree of the same name has a thin petiole and a profusion of small round scattered leaves. All types] cure lung fever.

tshar.bong: **Artemesia annua:** *Artemesia sieversiana* Willd: [is said to be a type of *mkhan.pa* and is of white, black and pale brown types. The brown type is a thick bush with many branches and has hot, bitter taste and strong odor. The white type also has strong odor, and all three types] cure throat fever and lung disorders.

tang.kun: a type of dill, **Peucedanum** sp. (white type): *Cnidium dahuricum: Chaerophyllum reflexum*: [is of two types. The white has long yellowish petioles, thin scattered leaves and a yellowish flower, with hot taste and pungent odor. The black type has leaves, stalk and root similar to *Angelica* and a yellow scented flower covered with black fur. Both types] cure heart fever, poisoning [and wind-phlegm combinations].

se.rgod: **Wild Rose** (female type): *Rosa macrophylla:* [is of superior and inferior sub-types and grows on very high hills]. Its rosehip cures liver fevers and fever caused by poisoning.

shug.pa.tsher.chan: **Sabina recurva** (Harriet) Antoine: *Juniperus recurva: Empetrum niger:* [has eight names and is of three types, *rgya.sung* (juniper), *lha.shug* and *shug.tsher*. It has a small, thorny trunk and] cures kidney fevers, infectious tissue degeneration, lymph disorders and heals wounds. The leaf is recommended for use in disorders of the lower intestine, whilst the fruit is said to be supreme in (curing) fever in the limbs, in drying lymph accumulations and as an essence-extraction ingredient.

skyer.pa: flower and fruit of **Indian Barberry:** *Berberis* *aristata* D.C.: *Berberis asiatica:* [has a yellow] flower and [reddish-blue] fruit which halts dysentery.

thang.phrom: **Thornapple:** *Datura stramonium: Datura alba* (white type) and *Anisodus luridus* Link et Otto: *Scopolia lurida*(black type): [has thirteen names, for example, *dha.du.ra,* and is of white and black types. It grows on high hills and rocky meadows. The white type has a thick green leaf, a thick dark red flower and a large seed pod. The black type grows on the plains and has a large stem, round green leaf, pale brown flower and seed pod. *Datura* has a hot taste, cures infectious tissue degeneration, sores and swellings and is also an aphrodisiac.]

lang.thang.tse: **Henbane:** *Hyoscyamus niger*Linn: [has nine names and grows in gardens. It has a tall, thin stalk, round (vase-) shaped pod containing sesame-like seeds, and a lobed green leaf]. Both *Datura* and henbane are anthelmintic.

srin.shing.na.ma: **Abutilon avicennae:** *Daphne odora: Stellaria media:* [has four names. It has silvery bark, scattered green leaves, long, flexible, brownish petioles, deep red flowers and bright red fruits which turn black after ripening. The inferior type has thin petioles, dark-green lobed leaves and white flowers]. The fruit of *Abutilon* has the same use as *Datura* [and increases digestive heat].

*dres.ma:***Iris ensata** Thumb: *Iris decora: Iris lactea* Pall.: [is of three types; the male type has two names, the female has three, and the neuter type has ten. The male type has thick linear leaves and a reddish-brown flower. The wild type has smaller fruit. The female type has a blue flower, a flexible leaf and is used to make ropes. The neuter type has an unattractive grey fruit and a reddish-blue flower]. Its petals are anthelmintic, relieve cramps, [neutralize poisons and are a general purgative].

dkar.po.chhig.thub. [One type is **Ginseng** (*Panax major* Burk., *Panax notoginseng* Burk.). It grows on cliffs and has a leaf and pod similar to *Datura*. It has a root similar to a dried radish, long thin petioles, and slender, flat green leaves. A second type has undulating leaves. The root of both types] collects poisons, heals septic disorders and is anthelmintic.

*a.wa:***Carex** sp.: *Lloydia serotina* Reichb.: [is of three types. It (is a grass with long, round, hollow, brittle stalks) which grow on north-facing rocks and has no flower, fruit or pod. The

inferior type, *a.wa.dar.dpyangs,* is threadlike and has no flower
or fruit, whereas both are found on the female type. All types]
are beneficial in chest sores and eye diseases, [and they
stimulate tooth growth and dispel spirits].

zhim.thig.le: **Geranium dahuricum:** *Plectranthus* sp. (black
type): *Geranium pratense: Euphrasia reqellii* Wettstein.:
Morrubium incisum: [has fifteen names. It has a square stem
with many joints, square petioles and a leaf similar to that of
nettle, but without sting. The flower is pale yellow and bitter
with black fruit. The black type has a coarse black leaf, square
hooded stalk, red flower and three-sided black seeds which
resemble cracked buckwheat. It has sweet taste and oily power.
The inferior type has a soft, glossy leaf, hard, square stalks,
brownish or bluish flowers and oily power. *Geranium* may also
have small, round, lobed leaves and five-petalled flowers. All
three main types] dispel cataract [as well as other eye diseases
and are anthelmintic].

par.pa.ta: **Common Fumitory:** *Fumaria officinalis* Linn:
Hypecoum leptocarpum Hook f. et Thoms: [has sixteen names.
It has green or blue leaves, a long thin stalk and a chickpea-
shaped berry. By its bitter taste and cool power, fumitory] cures
infectious fevers, fevers caused by poisoning [and bile fevers].

dva.wa: a type of **Typhonium giganteum** Engl.: *Arisaema
intermedium: Arisaema lobatum: Arisaema consanguineum:*
[has ten names and is of two types. The superior and wild type
grows on hills, whilst the common type grows in fields. It has
a thick, glossy leaf, pale yellow flower and fruits resembling a
mass of coral. *Typhonium* has hot taste and warm post-digestive power]. Its root is anthelmintic, removes bone excrescences [and cures swellings, sores and superfluous flesh
growths. The fruit is beneficial in cases of poisoning.]

hdam.bu.ka.ra: **Hippuris vulgaris:** *Juncus grisbachii:
Eleocharis palustris:* [grows in water and has a long, thin,
curling leaf. The superior type has sweet taste and cures bone
fever, punctured lung and brown phlegm. The inferior type
grows in ponds and has a leaf similar to that of onion. It has a
sweet taste and smooth power and cures bone fevers. The
different types of *Hippuris*] cure fevers of the lungs, liver and
channels.

hbri.ta.sa.hdzin: a type of **Wild Strawberry:** *Fragaria* *nilgeerensis* Schlecht: *Fragaria indica: Saxifraga flagellaris: Cuscuta europaea:* [has two names, for example, *glang*. It has small blue leaves, a red stalk, small pale yellow flowers, slightly sweet-tasting fruit and long runners]. *Fragaria* is an emetic in pus, blood and lymph disorders [as well as diseases in the upper body].

bya.po.tsi.tsi: **Celosia cristata** L.: *Goniolimon speciosum* L. Boiss: *Limonium (statice) flexuosum* L. (Rtze.): *Ceratostigma minus:* [has two names and resembles *ma.ma.sgo.lchags* and *lug.ru. smug.po.* It has a blue or yellowish-blue flower, red fruit and is also known as *bdud.rtse.aahu.rtsi* or *skyu.rug.ma.*] It controls excess menstrual flow, [is hemostatic, supremely beneficial for skull fractures and injuries, and unites bone fractures].

shu.mo.za: **Daucus carota:** *Trigonella foenum-graecum:* [has two names and grows in fields. It has a leaf and petals like that of the chickpea plant. The pod (fruit) resembles the foot of a chicken and the seed looks similar to a child's testicle]. It cures lung pus and diarrhoea.

snyi.wa: **Codonopsis convolvulacea** Kurz: *Fritillaria thunbergii:* [has seven names and is a climber similar to *Clematis*. It has a thin, green leaf and a bell-shaped flower similar to blue utpala. The root has predominantly sweet taste, improves appetite and sense of smell, and cures fevers of the channels and heart.]

lug.mur: **(Leucas) Phlomis kawaguchii** Murata: *Phlomis tuberosa:* [is also known as *pi.pi.lug.mur.* It has furry, yellowish-green leaves, square petioles and brown flowers. The fruit has sweet taste and cures lung disorders. Both *Codonopsis* and *Leucas*] cure chest fevers and common cold.

gyer.shing.pa: **Scrophularia incisa:** *Scrophularia ningpoensis* Hemsl: *Tournefortia sibirica:* [The superior type is dense and black, whereas the inferior type grows in damp areas and has a red petiole, yellow flower and seed similar to *Zanthoxylum (gyer.ma).*] It cures [all types of] pox-fever.

me.tog.ser.chhen: **Papaver nudicaule** L.: *Trollius asiaticus: Tagetes erecta* L.: [grows in dry soil and has a large, yellow flower, small, furry, lobed leaf, thin stalk and short petioles. It has bitter taste], unites wounds and heals necrosis of the channels.

brag.skya.ha.wo: **Corallodiscus Kingianus** (Craib) Burtt:
Dryopteris fragrans: Woodsia glabella: [has four names, for
example, *ming.po.bdun.gyi.sring.gchig.ma*(lit. 'single sister of
seven brothers') and *blon.po.re.ral* ('minister fern') and grows
beside rocks. It has a large, thick, stiff, lobed, flat leaf and a blue
flower which whitens with age. *Corallodiscus* has bitter and
sweet tastes], neutralizes poisons, halts dysentery with fever,
[heals wounds, kidney disorders and disorders of the seminal
vesicle].

brag.spos: **Lepisorus waltonii** ching: *Lepisorus
scolopendrium:* [has four names, for example, *btsun.mo.re.ral,*
etc. It has a swordlike, narrow, yellow leaf with four lobes at
the base covered with dewdrops. (At least two similar sub-
types have now been classified.)] *Lepisorus*heals wounds, dries
pus, sustains bone resin, [cures channel fevers and is beneficial
for injuries and enlargement of the diaphragm].

rgya.spos: **Melilotus suaveolens** ldb.: *Melilotus parviflora:*
[has ten names. It has long, thin petioles, yellow flower, sweet
fragrance, bitter taste and cool power.]

spangs.spos: **Indian Spikenard** or Muskroot: *Nardostachys
jatamansi* D.C.: [has twenty-five names and grows in shady
meadows. It has a brown stalk, turquoise leaf and extremely
fragrant red flower]. Both *Melilotus*and spikenard cure chronic
fever and fever caused by poisoning [and dispel spirits].

*myang.rtsi.spras*or *ser.po.khrag.rkang*or *lo.mar.sngo.sprin:*
Gold Thread: *Coptis teetoides: Adonis sibirica:* [has seven names.
It has a glossy, thin, lobed leaf, slender, flexible petioles and a
yellow, furry flower. Gold thread has bitter and astringent
tastes,], dries fluid [accumulations, pus, etc.], cures infectious
fever [and heals wounds. The inferior type is known as
sngo.sprin.khrag.rkang or *ldum.bu.lchags.kyu.chan*and has a
long, slightly yellow stalk, scattered green leaves and a slightly
bitter taste. Apart from a lack of fluid-drying properties it has
the same uses as the superior type above.]

rgud.drus: **Senecio scandens** Buch.Ham: *Senecio frabri L.:*
Galium boreale L.: [has a thin, smooth leaf, white flowers with
a reddish hue growing from each joint, and an ovary containing
seeds. It has hot and bitter tastes, and the flower may also be
pale blue and slightly yellow. The inferior type has a long,
slender, lobed leaf and yellow flower. Both types] heal wounds,

unite severed channels, cure colic [and wound fever, and are recommended in fever, infectious fever and poisoning].

hbam.po: **Meadow Sweet:** *Filipendula vestita* (Wall ex G. Don) Maxim: *Achillea setacea:* [has two names and grows around meadows. It has a leaf, flower and stalk similar to fennel, is malodorous and has a thick taste (i.e., phlegm-like or hard to distinguish). But for the fact that it has fewer leaves it would easily be mistaken for *rtsad.* The male type has a flower with stalk, whilst the female or black type lacks these. Both types] reduce swelling, remove internal abscesses (ulcers) [and glandular growths].

me.tog.lug.mig (lit. 'sheep's eye flower'):*Aster barbellatus: Aster heolini: Aster flaccidus* Bge.: [grows in rocky meadows and has small, rounded, pale blue leaves, tall, brown stalk and blue flowers with yellow pistils. It has slightly bitter taste, neutralizes] poison and cures contagious fevers.

mkhan.pa: **Mugwort:** *Artemesia sieversiana: Artemesia frigida: Artemesia vulgaris:* [has three names and is of three types. It is grey in appearance, has a fragrant yellow flower, small lobed leaf which grows close to the ground and is also known as *a.krong (dkar.mo).* It reduces swellings and is beneficial for wounds, abscesses and (disorders of) the large and small intestines. The white type has a thin petiole and pale blue leaf, whilst the red or brown type yields seeds,] is hemostatic and reduces swellings of the limbs. [The white sub-species is beneficial for kidney disorders and is recommended in essence-extraction compounds.]

chhu.ma.rtsi: a type of **Indian Rhubarb:** *Rheum nobile* Hook f. et Thoms: *Oxyria digyna* (mountain sorrel): *Polygonum polystachyum:* [is also known as *rtsi.stag.mo.* Some say it re-sembles a white bird on a perch, whilst others call it *mkhah.hgro.la.hphug,* and still others identify it as a hot tasting plant similar to *lchags.tig,* all of which are erroneous. It grows in muddy areas and fields. The superior or black type has a bluish-green, lanceolate leaf, red inflorescence and red peti-oles. The white type has long, green petioles, a sword-shaped leaf, a pink flower which leaves behind a straight seed pod, and bitter taste. Both types] purge lymph (accumulations) and oedema.

byi.tsher: Fagonia cretica Linn: *Xanthium sibiricum* Patr.:

Xanthium strumarium: [has three names and grows in sandy areas. It has a small, dark, thick leaf, short, thick, hard, dark yellowish-green stalk and burrs which stick to one's clothes. *Fagonia* has bitter taste, coarse power,] cures infectious fever, poisoning, kidney fever [and relieves urinary retention].

de.wa: Primula sibirica Jaqueum (herb): **Populus alba:** *Populus bonatii* (tree): [has four names. The *de.wa* herb has a dark blue flower, grows to a height of four finger-breadths, and the inferior type has a thick leaf. The *de.wa* tree has a whitish bark and many hard knots in the trunk]. It cures infectious fevers [and shooting pains].

rtsa.mkhris: Ixeris gracilis D.C.: *Cierhita macrorhiza: Sonchus* sp.: [has two names. It has a yellow, four-petalled flower, coarse green leaf similar to that of dandelion and milky sap]. Ixeris cures bile disorders.

re.ral: a type of **Fern:** *Adiantum pedatum* L.: *Adiantum aspidium:* [has five names, for example *rgyal.po.re.ral*(lit. 'king fern') and *ldum.bu.re.ral*. It grows on the trunks of trees, and has a furry root similar to a monkey's tail, slightly sweet taste, cool power and the shape of the leaf is similar to a tongue of flame.]

ldum.bu.re.ral: Drynaria propinqua: Polystichum squarrosum: is said to be the 'king fern', whilst *brags.spos (Lepisorus)* is the 'queen fern' and *brags.skya.ha.wo (Corallodiscus)* is the 'minister fern'].

hom.bu or *chhu.shing.hom.bu:* **Tibetan Tamarisk:** *Myricaria germanica* Beaucv.: *Myricaria prostrata:* [has six names and grows on river banks and in sandy areas. It has a tall brown stalk, clusters of reddish-brown flowers, a thin green leaf and bitter-sweet taste]. *Adiantum* and *Myricaria* neutralize meat poison and compounded poison [and cure bile fevers. The external application of *Myricaria* is beneficial for *sur.ya* sores.[16]]

zhu.mkhan: leaf of the **Lodh Tree:** *Symplocos racemosa* Roxb.: *Symplocos paniculata: Symplocos crataegoides:* [has fifteen names, for example *seng.phrom,* etc. The superior type has a large trunk, a large thick, yellowish-green leaf and is known as *spang.zhun.* The inferior type is known as *nags.zhun* and has a dark green leaf.]

tshos: **Bastard Teak:** *Butea monosperma* (Lam.) Kuntze:

Lithospermum officinale var. erythrorhizon: *Laccifer lacea*
Kerr.: [has eight names, for example *rgya.skyegs* or *ke.shu.ka*
tree. The flowers are internally red with yellow pistils and black
underside to the petals. According to seasonal influence the
resin is of two types, known as *dro.tsho* and *nag.hrug*]

btsod: **Indian Madder** or Dyer's Madder: *Rubia cordifolia*
Linn.: *Rubia tinctorium:* [has thirteen names and is a climber
which also spreads on the ground. It has a green leaf and thin
petioles. Lodh, bastard teak and madder] cure spreading fever
of the lungs and kidneys.

lcham.pa: a type of **Mallow:** *Malva verticillata* Linn:
Dalbergia lanceolaria: [has six names, for example *nyi.dgah*
(name of the neuter type) and *phor.mdog.ldan.* The male type
is known as *ha.mdog.ldan.* It has a long petiole, blue leaf and
white or pale brown flower. The female type is known as
rgya.lcham.pa and has a round leaf, thin, long petiole and
white or pale brown flower. *Nyi.dgah,* the neuter type, is also
called *a.dza.ka,* i.e. the former name refers to the leaf and the
latter one to the seed. It has sweet and astringent tastes], cures
urinary retention, diarrhea, [kidney fever, quenches] thirst [and
dries wound pus. The male type, or *ha.lchi.me.tog* (flower), halts
nocturnal emission, whilst the root, known as *pa.la,* is beneficial in consumption and anorexia.]

brag.lcham: **Bergenia ciliata:** *Pyrola rotundifolia: Pyrola
incarnata:* [grows on rocks. It has a thick round, glossy, green
leaf with dewdrops and a red or white flower. This plant] heals
wounds.

rta.rmig (lit. 'horse's hoof'): **Epimedium grandiflorum:**
Aristolochia contorta: Asarum heterotropoides: Viola biflora:
[grows at the base of rocks. It has a lobed leaf and yellow
flower, and both leaf and flower are shaped like a horse's hoof.
In the absence of stalk and branches the leaf grows straight
from the ground (sessile growth)]. *Epimedium* constricts the
openings of the channels.

gra.ma: **Caragana franchetia** Kom: *Caragana brevifolia:
Caragana pygmaea:* [is a thorny bush with a dull yellow flower
and white wood separated by a gap from the bark. It has bitter
taste, cool power, and its] root cures flesh- and channel-fevers.

mdzo.mo: **Caragana jubata** Poir: *Caragana gerardiana:*
[is a thorny tree, larger than *gra.ma* and covered with white

'fur'. It has a yellow flower and heartwood similar to red sandalwood.] *Caragana* dissolves blood clots and cures blood fever.

phang.ma: **Eleagnus pungens:** *Lycium barbarum: Lycium chinense: Leonurus heterophyllus* Sweet: [has thin leaves and a pale trunk from which the branches protrude horizontally. It has a sweet-tasting reddish-brown] seed, [which is of two types, black and white, and] cures heart fevers and gynecological disorders.

srad.dkar.wa: type of **Gum Tragacanth:** *Astragalus yunnaneansis: Oxytropis oxyphylla:* [has ten names and is of three types, white, black and *byehu.srad.ma.* The superior or white type grows in sandy areas, has a white, furry leaf and stalk and a bright white flower which cures phlegm disorders. The common type has a bluish hue and] purges first and third stages of oedema. [*byehu.srad.ma*] has a leaf and flower similar to the above types, a pouch-like seed-pod, small, hard seeds and dries lymph [accumulations].

byi.rug: **Elscholtzia** sp.: [is said to be of yellow and black types (black type: *Elscholtzia calycocarpa; Stachys baicalensis*). The superior type has thin, flexible petioles, an elongated, green leaf, an inflorescence similar to a golden stupa and a pungent smell. The types with black, or yellowish-black ears have round leaves. All three types have hot and astringent tastes and] heal wounds and sores infected by parasites, worms, etc.

mtshe.ldum: **Ephedra saxatilis** Royle: *Ephedra intermedia: Ephedra sinica* Stapf.: [has two names and is a type of jointed grass growing in rocky areas. It is green with red flowers and rounded petals and grows about fifteen centimeters high. The *lug.mtshe* type is seed-bearing, whilst *ra.mtshe* has no seed]. *Ephedra* [has bitter taste and] stops bleeding from the veins and arteries, cures liver fever, [is an expectorant, disperses tumors, reduces swellings and is a recommended ingredient in essence-extraction compounds].

bre.ga: **Thlaspi arvense** Linn.: *Ailanthus glandulosa:* [has four names and grows in fields and fertile areas. It has an arrow-like stalk, drum-like seed-pod, thick, bright, green leaf and black sesame-like seeds. *Thlaspi* has bitter taste, oily power and] cures lung and kidney fevers, and [single phlegm and lymph disorders].

lug.chhung: **Aster diplostaphioides** (D.C.) C.B. Clarke:
Aster strachei: Aster poliothamnus: [has three names. It is
slightly furry, has a pale blue flower, and its leaf and stalk
resemble *Aster flaccidus (lug.mig)*]. It cures infectious fevers,
poisoning, brown phlegm and channel fevers. [This type of
Aster is also malodorous, has bitter taste and cool power,
disperses spirits and (heals) infected wounds.]

*lug.ngal:***Corydalis meifolia:** *Linaria buriatica:* [the white
type grows on river banks and has a soft leaf and thin petiole.
It is adhesive, with a green leaf and pale yellow flower.
Corydalis has a sweet taste and cool power,] neutralizes
poisons, reduces swellings of the limbs [and is outstanding in
relieving pain caused by wind imbalances].

zangs.rtsi.wa: **Galium spurium** Linn: *Galium aparine* L.:
Artemesia scoparia (white type): [has three names. The white
type has a thin, square petiole and seed which adheres to
clothing and helps to produce curd when boiled in milk. It also
has red pods containing small, black seeds. The black type
grows in dark soft soil and has a strong smell similar to
mkhan.pa (Artemesia)]. It cures jaundice and (all types of) bile
disorders. [The leaf of the latter type is also said to be beneficial
in sinusitis.]

rnya.lo or *snya.lo:* **Polygonum hydropiper:** *Polygonum
periginatoris*Pauls: *Polygonum companulatum:* [grows on shady
hills. It has a coarse leaf, long, red, flexible stalk and dense
clusters of white flowers. It has sour and slightly bitter taste and]
cures fevers of the large and small intestines and vessel organs
[abdominal disorders and chronic diseases].

sho.mang: **Dockleaf:** *Rumex hepatonsis* Spr.: *Rumex
nepalensis: Rumex acetosa:* [has three names and is generally
classified according to five types, i.e., hill dock (*ri.sho;* see below),
sheep dock (*lug.sho*) and plains dock (*klung.sho*). It has a large,
red, jointed stalk, a large, glossy, flat, smooth, green leaf and
coarse red or yellow flowers. It has sweet and bitter tastes.
Chhu.sho('waterdock') is also called *ga.bra.ma* or *chhu.sha.wa.*
It is smaller than the above type, has slightly sour taste and no
stalk]. Dockleaf cures wound fevers [and is beneficial in
infectious fevers].

*pa.yag:***Lancea tibetica:** *Salvia miltiorrhiza: Viola dissecta:*
[has ten names. The leaves grow close to the ground, and it has

a blue flower with a tinge of red and a seed in the shape of an animal's heart. It is also known as *gyag.snying.lug.(snying)* and *bya.rog.nor.bu*]. The root of *pa.yag* [has sweet and slightly bitter tastes], heals lung diseases, drains lung pus [and disperses womb tumors].

*bye.bu.la.phug: **Malcolmia africana*** (L.) R.Br.: *Dontostemon pectinatus: Draba alata:* [has two names and grows in marshes. It has a narrow, thick green leaf, white flower and grows about fifteen centimeters high; one type tastes like radish. Both superior and inferior types] cure meat poisoning [and indigestion].

*aoog.chos: **Incarvillea youngbusbandii:*** *Incarvillea compacta* Maxim: *Gossipium herbaceum: Paeonia anomala:* [has a red, yellow or white flower. The red type grows on rocks or cliffs. It has lobed leaves lying close to the ground, flowers similar to bunches of coral that contain vajra-like pistils, and seed-pods shaped like the curved horns of a wild sheep that contain leguminous seeds. *Incarvillea* has bitter and sweet tastes], cures ear diseases, purges swellings [and is carminative].

*skyi.wa: **Sophora moorcroftiana*** (Wall) Benth ex. Baker: [is also known as *ngang.pa.gchig.rgyug.dar.ya.kan.* It is a grey, thorny bush, with a small, thin leaf, pale blue flower and rectangular pod containing red seeds. *Sophora* is fragrant with bitter taste and its] seed is a bile emetic. [It is also anthelmintic and treats diphtheria and quinsy.]

Sardzika: **Corn Smut:** *Ustilago* sp.: [has eight names, for example *skyi.snye* and is a black fungus which grows on ears of corn]. It increases digestive heat [and is beneficial for wounds].

*srub.ka: **Anemone rivularis*** Buch-Ham: *Pulsatilla patens: Ranunculus:* [has five names, for example *ra.srub, rgyal.po.tso.ra,* etc. It has a flexible petiole, rounded, smooth tri-segmented leaf, a dull pale blue or white flower and a stalk which splits into four parts. *Anemone* has hot and bitter tastes], halts necrosis, increases digestive heat, drains lymph [accumulations and removes cold tumors].

*lche.tsha: **Ranunculus acris:*** *Ranunculus pulchellus:* [has six names, for example *ser.hdab.lnga.pa, bong.bu.lan.tshra,* etc., and grows in shady meadows. The superior or female type has a lobed, rough, pale green leaf and a large, yellow five-petalled flower. The inferior or male type has a large, thick leaf shaped like a frog's foot.] *Ranunculus* removes cold tumors, diphtheria and quinsy, etc., and dries oedema fluid.

dbyi.mong: **Clematis montana** Buch-Ham: *Clematis alpina* (white type): [has fourteen names, for example *a.za.mo, rlung.ni.brla.reng.dus, rtsa.bya,* etc., and is of black and white types. It is a climbing (shrub) with a coarse, dark-green leaf and a dull, white bell-shaped flower. It has hot and slightly sweet taste and removes tumors. The white, yellow-tinted *Clematis* is asserted to be *khra.wo* and is most inferior in quality. The black type, also known as *za.byed.nag.po.khar,* has a dark slightly coarse leaf and a dark flower]. *Ranunculus* and *Clematis* both have the same use as *Anemone.*

ba.lu: **Rhododendron anthopogonoides:** *Rhododendron affcephalanthum* (white type): [has three names, for example *(bdud.rtsi.)da.li* (name of the flower of the white type) grows on high shady hills. It has a white stem, blue leaf and a white or dark flower. The white type has sweet, bitter and astringent tastes and smooth power]. *da.li* cures phlegm disorders, hot and cold reactive conditions, [lung diseases, first stage oedema and hoarseness caused by any of the three humors, and is a recommended ingredient in essence-extraction compounds].

go.snyod: **Fennel:** *Foeniculum vulgare: Carum carvi:* [has five names. It has a flat, elongated, lobed leaf, a tall, thin stalk, thin petiole and white umbelliferous flower]. Fennel cures wind fevers, poisoning, eye diseases, [and phlegm disorders, reduces swelling and improves appetite].

tha.ram: **Plantago depressa** Willd: *Plantago major vulgaris latifolia* var. *asiatica:* [has four names, for example *be.khur,* and grows in fields and by the roadside. It has a glossy, green lobed leaf, grows tall and erect, has a green petiole and a green inflorescence. One sub-species has a pale green leaf, a yellow multiple flower and is without petiole.] *Plantago* has sweet and astringent tastes, heals wounds and dries lymph accumulations.

na.ram: **Polygonum alopecuroides:** *Polygonum viviparum:* [has three names, for example *ram.bu* and *skam.rtsi.* It grows on shady hills and plains and has an elongated, green leaf, greyish flower similar to a dog's tail, small red seed and a glossy red root.]

bya.rkang (lit. 'bird's foot,' referring to the shape of the leaf):

Larkspur: *Delphinium grandiflorum: Delphinium viscosum:* [has nine names, for example, *ti.mu.sa, chhe.war.lo.btsan, rma.lo.rkang.gchig* and *sngon.mo.dar.ya.kan.* It has a tall thin stalk, a slightly blue leaf, a reddish-blue flower shaped like the head of a hoopoe bird, and long, thin, green petioles. Larkspur has slightly bitter taste, halts dysentery and] is beneficial against external parasites, lice, etc. *Plantago, Polygonum alopecuroides* and larkspur halt diarrhea.

sog.ka.pa: **Shepherd's Purse:** *Capsella bursa* Pastoris (L.) Medic.: [has five names. It has a small white flower and stalk, a small (wavy-edged) leaf and a triangular seed-(case containing tiny yellow seeds)]. Shepherd's purse stops all forms of vomiting.

dwang.po.lag.pa: a type of **Salep Orchid:** *Orchis incarnata* Linn.: [has twelve names, for example *brgya.bying,* etc., and grows in meadows and near springs. Its root resembles a man's hand (i.e., with five-fingered tubers), and the flowers are yellowish-blue. It has a green leaf and petiole and an inflorescence resembling the layered structure of a stupa. The six-fingered type is known as *tsogs.bdag* (Ganesh), whilst the five-fingered type is known as *sbang.lag* (Indrahanta), the four-fingered type as *dri.zahi.lag.pa* (Gandhamadna) and the single tuber as *thehu.rang.* The common type has a yellow flower, and all types having three or more tubers] are tonic, aphrodisiac [and collect poison].

ri.sho: **Hill Dockleaf:** *Rumex crispus: Ligularia laesicotal* Kitam: *Ligularia achyrotricha:* [has seven names, for example *shehu.sga.dar,* etc. It has a large leaf, coarse stalk, yellow flower, seed similar to that of lotus and is of two types according to size. Hill dock has sweet and bitter tastes, cool post-digestive power and] is a bile- [and phlegm-] emetic. It also heals wounds and chronic infectious fevers.

sbyang.tsher or *spyang.tsher:* a type of **Thistle:** *Cirsium* sp.: *Morina betanicoides: Echinops* sp.: [has three names and is of black and white types. The superior white type grows in shady, dark soil and has thorny, lobed leaves spreading close to the ground. It has a tall, flexible stalk and tassel-like flower. The black type has a green leaf similar to the above type and a mauve flower. The inferior white type is without petiole and has a flower growing from the center of the leaf]. Thistle is a phlegm emetic [and heals wounds and sores].

dur.byid: **Jatropha glandulifera:** *Baliospermum montanum* (Physic Nut): *Iris dichotoma: Euphorbia adenochlora: Euphorbia fischeriana:* [has ten names, for example *tri.byi.ta.* It has a single root, horizontally protruding petioles, a green leaf, reddish-brown four-petalled flower, and rounded, three-sided fruit. The inferior type is without fruit].

thar.nu: **Euphorbia pallassii:** *Baliospermum sinulatum: Euphorbia wallichiana: Croton tiglium:* [has eight names. It has a thick, heavy stalk and taproot, and red flower, petiole and seed. Euphorbia has hot taste, removes stones and pustules and in calcinated form is anti-emetic.] *Jatropha* and *Euphorbia* purge all hot and cold disorders.

*sngon.bu:***Lactuca dissecta:** *Lactuca dolichophylla: Lactuca lessertiana:* [has four names and is said to be a tree from which paper is produced. (However) it grows in high meadows, has a green, furry leaf which spreads on the ground, a blue bell-shaped flower with a reddish tint, and milky sap]. *Lactuca* purges lymph disorders.

*khron.bu:***Physalis peruviana:** *Clerodendron fortunatum: Euphorbia sieboldiana* [has three names. It has a small, round green leaf and a taproot and] purges bile disorders.

lchum.rtsa: **Indian Rhubarb:** *Rheum emodi* Wall: *Rheum webbianum: Rheum palmatum:* [has eleven names, for example *zhim.shing, rtsa.wa.shing,* etc. It grows in rocky areas and is of large, medium and small types. Its green leaf spreads close to the ground, whilst the stalk is tall, hollow and flexible. The flower is red or yellow, with a three-sided seed which cures phlegm disorders. Indian Rhubarb has sour taste and coarse power], and purges fever caused by poisoning, vessel organ fever and phlegm disorders.

chhu.rtsa: **Rheum spiciforme:** *Rheum officinale:* [has seven names. The male type has a hollow petiole, large, thick, green leaf, known as *tha.chhu.ra,* and a yellow, three-sided ear, or fruit. The female type has a red, solid petiole, small inflorescence and a leaf similar to the above, known as *rdza.chhu.rar.* The neuter type is of two (sub-species, one of which has a large leaf and short petiole, whilst the other has a short, red petiole and hard leaf)]. *Rheum* purges septic conditions, dries [accumulations of] fluid in wounds, [cures phlegm disorders and brown phlegm, and acts as a test for poison].

re.lchag.pa: ***Stellera chamaejasme*** L.: [has four names. It has a single root, thick, glossy, sessile leaf and bright red flower. *Stellera* has hot taste and coarse power], heals sores, purges septic disorders [and is used as a suppository].

lcha.wa: ***Angelica archangelica:*** *Angelica dahurica: Polygonatum odoratum* (Mill) Druce var. *pluriflorum:* [has nine names, for example *stong.nag,* and grows on shady hills. The superior type has a leaf similar to a turquoise mandala, a white umbel flower and brown stalk. The common type has a brown stalk, white flower and is favored among the 'Five Roots.' Both types have hot, bitter and sweet tastes and] cure lymph disorders, cold disorders of the waist and kidneys, [cold phlegm diseases, stomach disorders, first stage oedema and wind diseases. *ba.lang.lcha.wa* has appearance and uses similar to the common type above. Applied as a fomentation it is beneficial in swellings and distention.]

nye.shing: ***Asparagus filicinus:*** *Asparagus racemosus* Willd: *Polygonatum falcatum:* [has eighteen names. It has a tall, thin, thorny stalk and a seed resembling an iron pea. The root has bitter and astringent tastes and] cures disorders of the xiphoid process.

ra.mnye: ***Polygonatum verticillatum:*** *Polygonatum cathcartii: Polygonatum officinale: Polygonatum cirrifolium* (Wall) Royle: [has eighteen names and grows in isolated areas. It has a pale, yellow spreading root, green sword-like leaf, red flower and small seeds. *Polygonatum* has sweet, bitter and astringent tastes, cures wind disorders and first stage oedema, is highly recommended in essence-extraction compounds and is supreme among the 'Five Roots']. Both *Asparagus racemosus* and *Polygonatum* promote longevity and cure lymph disorders.

a.sho.gandha: **Winter Cherry:** *Withania somnifera* Dunal: *Physalis flexuosa* Linn.: *Asparagus lucidus:* [has seven names, for example, *ba.spru.wa.* The Sanskrit name (above) means 'horse smell.' It grows on the Indian plains and is of white and red flowering types. The white type has a round, sticky, pale green leaf with thin petiole, whilst the red type has an attractive pale flower. Winter cherry has hot and sweet tastes], cures cold disorders of the lower body, lymph disorders, [wind disorders, and first stage oedema, and dissolves calculi. The dark flowered type is not suitable for use in medicine.]

gze.ma: **Small Caltrops:** *Tribulus terrestris* Linn.: [has nine names and grows in desert areas. It has spreading leaves and stalk, a small, pale yellow flower, thorny (star-shaped) seed and may be classified according to five or eight types. Caltrops has sweet taste], cures urinary retention, rheumatism, kidney disorders, all types of wind disorders, first and second stages of oedema and *glang.shu,* (a skin disease similar to scabies).

(5) Medicines of Animal Origin

The thirteen medicines of animal origin consist of horn, bone, meat, blood, bile, fat, brain, skin, nails, hair, urine, droppings and whole body. Their indications and powers are explained as follows:

Horn

bse.ru: **Rhino:** [has four names and is of three colors, white, variegated and black in descending order of quality]. It dries [accumulations of] pus, blood and lymph in the stomach [and is beneficial in cases of poisoning].

kha.sha: **Spotted Deer:** *Capreolus capreolus* L.: [has two names. It has bulky horns approximately fifteen centimeters long].

sha.wa: **Tibetan Deer:** *Cervus elaphus:* [has three names]. The horns [of these two types of deer have] similar [action] to Rhino horn.

gtsod: **Hodgson's Antelope:** *Pantholops hodgsoni:* [has seven names. It heals wounds and is oxytocic (facilitates childbirth)].

dgo.wa: **Procapra pictaudata** Hodgson v. Hook: *Prodorcas gutturosa:* [has nine names. It dries pus (accumulations) in the abdomen]. The horn of Hodgson's antelope and Procapra halt diarrhoea.

rgya: **Saiga Antelope:** *Saiga tatarica: Nemorhaedus cripus:* [has six names. It has slender, black, very finely pleated horns].

thug: **Ram:** [has nine names]. The horns of Ram and Saiga antelope are ecbolic.

rgod.gyag: **Takin:** Wild yak: *Budorcas taxicolor:* [has ten names and is also known as *hbrong*]. Its horn increases [body] heat, disperses tumors, [and dries (accumulations of) pus in the abdomen].

gnyan: **Wild Sheep:** *Ovis ammon:* [has thirteen names. Its horn is shaped like that of a ram but is larger and] cures infectious fevers.

Bone

Human skull from a cemetery: dries lymph (accumulations).

Human bone: [is beneficial in heart diseases]. If the bone is a weather beaten scapula [shoulder-blade] in ash form it removes stubborn, chronic fever.

Human hip bone: removes infectious tissue degeneration.

Dragon bone: [has sixteen names]. It halts necrosis and heals glandular growths.

Tiger bone: [has fifteen names]. It increases bone resin.

hgron.bu: **Cowrie shell:** [has eight names, for example *karshapani* etc.] It is hemostatic, dries pus, [oedema fluid and lymph (accumulations), disperses tumors and is beneficial in eye diseases].

The bones of those killed by thunderbolts and the skull-bone of colic victim: cures colic.

Pig bone: [has nine names, for example *gtig.mug.*] It cures brown phlegm.

Sheep bone: cures (all types of) wind disorders. Bone from the head of a sheep's femur (thigh bone) dispels urinary retention.

zer.mo: **Porcupine bone:** *Pucrasia macrolopha:* [has six names and] is hemostatic.

spre.hu: **Monkey bone:** [has seven names. It is ecbolic [and abortifacient].

hbu.skyog: **Snail:** *Cipangopaludina chinensis* Gray: [has ten names. Its shell] is anthelmintic and purges oedema fluid.

bshul.chhags: **bone of Packhorse/Mule:** cures lymph disorders.

Meat

Human flesh: [also known as *sha.chen,* lit. 'great flesh'] heals sores, cures wind disorders, poisoning and septic conditions.

Snake meat: *Elaphe dione* (Pallas): [has eleven names, for example *kluhi.sha*]. It removes growths, dispels urinary retention, is beneficial in eye disorders, [painful fevers in children, lung diseases, leprosy and infected wounds, and it heals bone warts].

Vulture meat: [has fourteen names]. It increases [digestive] heat, removes goiters [and dispels spirits].

Peacock meat: [has seventeen names]. It subdues bile disorders, poisoning [and spirits]. (Peacock's feather is highly recommended as a test for poisoning. The feather should be swallowed in the evening, removed from the stool next day and washed. If the feather has undergone no discoloration the presence of poison is clearly indicated; however, if discoloration has taken place, then some other type of disease is present).

da.pyid: **Male White Snow Frog:** *Phrynosoma* sp.: [has nine names, for example *phuhi.rgyal.po.*] Its flesh cures cold disorders of the waist and kidneys. [Its urine is a highly recommended aphrodisiac].

sram: **Otter:** *Lutra lutra* L.: [has eight names]. Its liver cures urinary retention.

hphyi.wa: **Marmot:** *Marmota bobak* Muller: *Marmota himalayana* Hodgson: [has seven names]. Its liver unites cracks [and fractures] in bones.

Goat liver: [has nine names]. It is supremely beneficial in eye diseases [and as an anthelmintic].

The lungs, heart, liver, spleen, kidneys and flesh (of various animals) cure diseases of those respective organs.

shyang.kihi.pho.wa: **Wolf's stomach:** [has twelve names] It increases digestive heat and digests undigested food, [especially meat]. Its tongue removes swellings of the tongue.

Pig tongue: removes bone warts.

Dog tongue: [has ten names and] heals all types of wounds.

Donkey tongue: [has fourteen names]. It halts diarrhoea.

thug.hbras: **Ram testicle:** is aphrodisiac.

Dog testicle: is ecbolic.

Lungs of fox (*wa*) and of *khug.rta:* **Cuculus melanoleucus:** *Riparia riparia: Hirundo rustica:* (a type of swallow): heal punctured lungs.

bya.wang.sha: **Bat flesh:** [has thirteen names]. It is antiemetic [and dispels spirits].

mchhil.pa: **Sparrow:** *Passer montanus:* [has seven names].

nas.zan bird (lit. 'barley feeder'): **Asian sparrow:** [has ten names].

rtsangs.pa: a type of **Gecko:** *Agama himalayana sacra:* [has eleven names, for example *sder.chhags*. The flesh of] these three creatures increases semen, [is aphrodisiac, tonic and anodyne, and drains pus.]

ngur.pa: **Red Wild Duck:** *Anas nyroca: Tadorna ferruginea* (Pallas.) [has fourteen names, for example, *bande,* etc.] Its flesh cures anterior transposition of the calf muscle.

Blood

sha.wahi.khrag: **Deer blood:** is anthelmintic, halts bleeding from the womb [and prevents hangovers.]

Goat blood: cures venereal diseases, smallpox, [brown phlegm and leprosy].

The blood of wild yak and of Hodgson's antelope (*gtsod*): halts diarrhoea.

Pig blood: collects [scattered types of] poisoning and brown phlegm.

Donkey blood: cures rheumatism and lymph disorders in the joints.

bya.(tsha.lu.)yi.ze.khrag: **Rooster's comb blood:** [has fifteen names]. It stimulates flesh growth, maintains bone resin [and cures anterior transposition of the calf muscle.]

Womb blood: constricts the mouths of the channels, regenerates flesh [around wounds, and is beneficial for warts].

Bile

All the various types of bile constrict the mouths of the channels, halt necrosis, stimulate flesh growth, neutralize poison and are beneficial in eye disorders.

Fat

Snake fat: expels bullets, (shrapnel, etc.) [and cures anterior transposition of the calf muscle.]

Deer fat: is anthelmintic and protects against poisoning.

Pig fat: collects poison, heals psoriasis [and cures baldness].

Human fat: subdues wind disorders and heals psoriasis.

Brain

Goat brain: unites severed ligaments and tendons.

Sheep brain: cures dizziness and vertigo.

Brain of game animals (e.g. deer): halts diarrhoea.

Rabbit brain: cures colic.
Human brain: reduces swellings and cures lymph disorders.

Skin
   Snake skin: cures leucoderma, *glang.shu* (a skin disease) [and is beneficial against *bhuta*-spirits[17]].
   Rhino hide and **Ox hide:** cure smallpox.
   Rat and Mouse skin: drains all types of pus accumulations.

Nails
   Crocodile: [has twenty-two names]. Its claw cures bone fevers. If crocodile claw is not obtainable one should use *na.gi,* which is an ingredient in compounded incense.
   bong.buhi.rmig.pa: the (right) hoof of (a one-year-old black) **Donkey:** cures urinary retention [and infectious fevers].
   Horse's hoof: removes tumors [and is beneficial against nagas].
   Horse's ankle bone: cures anterior transposition of the calf muscle [and subdues nagas].

Hair
   Crown feather of peacock: cures poisoning, pus accumulation in the lungs, [and ear diseases, and subdues nagas].
   so.bya: **Heron:** *Larus canus Kamtschatschensis: Phalacrocorax carbo sinensis:* [has fourteen names]. Its feathers relieve urinary retention [and dispel spirits].
   hug.pa: **Owl:** [has fifteen names]. Its feather cures oedema.
   bya.ma.byi: **Fruit Bat:** *Vespertilio superans:* [has sixteen names]. Its [tail] feathers expel womb disorders.
   gnah.wa: **Burrhel sheep:** *Ovis nahur: Rupicapra rupicapra:* Chamois: *Pseudo nayaur* Hodgson: [has eight names]. Its fur neutralizes poison.
   ra.thug.rmongs.spus: **Pubic hair of billy-goat:** cures infectious tissue degeneration.

Urine
   Human urine: cures septic disorders, is anthelmintic and is prophylactic against infectious fevers.
   Cow urine (especially that of the superior red-brown cow): purges lymph disorders and chronic fevers.

Droppings
Vulture's droppings: increase digestive heat, disperse tumors and suppurate swellings.

Pig's stool: cures indigestion, septic disorders, infectious fevers and bile tumors.

Human excreta: cure gall stones, neutralize poisons, reduce swellings [and subdue spirits].

Horse dung: is anthelmintic, anti-emetic, cures wind-bile combinations [and is beneficial against spirits].

Rabbit droppings: purge oedema [and are beneficial for wounds].

Dog stool: [is especially beneficial against spirits].

Wolf stool and droppings of *Gong.mo:* **Tetragallus bimalayensis:** [all three] reduce swellings.

Bird and Rat droppings: both drain pus [accumulations].

phug.ron: **Pigeon droppings:** *Columba rupestris rupestris* Pallas: suppurate swellings [and, as a fomentation, are beneficial in phlegm disorders and 'white' rheumatism].

byang.pa: **Beetle:** *Mylabris phalerata: Mylabris cichorii* Fabricius: [has four names]. It purges all channel disorders.

Crab: [has nine names], and *chhu.sbur:* **Tibetan ant:** Both dispel urinary retention. (Tibetan ant in particular is a mild purgative of channel disorders).

bse.sbur: **Tibetan cockroach:** *Blatta orientalis* L.: *Periplaneta americana: Geotrupes laevistriatus:* (a large, black, malodorous, nocturnal insect): [is beneficial in septic fevers and for *lte.mkhad,* a children's disease].

bying.bying.thu.lus: **Dung beetle** and **Scarab beetle:** both types found under dung: [has five names and relieves urinary retention. These two types of insect] and Tibetan cockroach are anti-spasmodic.

spru.mahi.hbu: **Moxa insect: Chrysalis:** (a long insect found on crops): stops bleeding from the veins [or arteries].

na.bun.bu.mo: **Slug:** [has eight names] and stops discharge of sinus fluid.

chhu.byi (colloquial *chhu.yer*): **Water rat** (amphibious rodent with long snout and tail):

rba.byi: **Cinclus cinclus** (a white-throated aquatic bird): Its flesh and that of water rat cure meat poisoning.

rmigs.pa: **Eremias argus:** *Phrynocephalus vlangalii* Strauch:[has nine names, is] anthelmintic and neutralizes poisons.

Medicinal horses (i.e., the vehicle or base for compounded ingredients) include raw cane sugar, the horse for curing cold and wind disorders; crystal sugar, the horse for curing disorders of the blood, bile and fevers; and honey, the horse for curing lymph and phlegm disorders.

Thus the powers of the individual medicines (have been expounded), and it is important, that (you) sages retain them (in your minds).

This concludes the twentieth chapter, on the powers of medicines, from *The Quintessence Tantra, the Secret Oral Tradition of the Eight Branches of the Science of Healing.*

21. The Principles of Medicines: Compounding of Medicines

Then the Sage Rig.pahi.ye.she spoke these words: O Great Sage, listen. The compounding [of medicines entails the two] classes of [medicines] compounded [according to] taste, and those compounded [according to] power. Categories of medicines which cure diseases are shown (as follows):

The category of medicines that are standard cures for fevers includes Camphor, White Sandalwood, Bile of elephant and so forth, Bamboo concretion, Saffron and Blue Lily.

The class of medicines which cure bile disorders includes Chiretta, Bitter Cucumber, Kurchi bark, White Aconite, *Ixeris gracilis*, *Pyrola incarnata*, *Gentiana straminea* and Indian Barberry.

The class of medicines which cure blood disorders consists of Red Sandalwood, *Caragana jubata*, Catechu tree, *Picrorhiza*, Vasaka (Malabar Nut tree), Emblic Myrobalan, *Corydalis edulis*, *Pterocephalus hookeri*, Madder and Bastard Teak.

The categories of medicines which cure infectious fevers includes Bile of elephant and so forth, Bitter Cucumber, White Aconite, Meadow Cranesbill (*Geranium pratense*), *Fagonia cretica*, *Populus alba* (tree), *Primula sibirica* (herb), Common Fumitory and Gold Thread.

The class of medicines which neutralize poisons consists of Musk, Red, Yellow and White Aconites, White and Brown *Uncaria*, (white) *Phytolacca esculenta* (var. Houtte), (a type of Pokeberry), (yellow) *Scutellaria baicalensis, Pleurospermum hookeri, Senecio dianthus, Scutellaria, Oxytropis chiliophylla, Corallodiscus kingianus,* Turmeric, *Gentiana urnula,* Fern, Tibetan tamarisk, *Gentiana algida, Pterocephalus hookeri,* Wild Rose and the cambium (middle bark) of Indian Barberry.

The category of medicines for lung disorders includes Bamboo concretion, Liquorice, Raisin, *Hippophae rhamnoides,* Costus root, Meadow Cranesbill (*Geranium pratense*), *Gypsophila dahurica (Artemesia), Cochlearia scapiflora* and *Solms-Laubachia.*

The class of medicines used in wind fevers includes Heart-leaved Moonseed, Indian Salamin, Eaglewood, Fennel, Costus root, Black Sal resin and Garlic.

The category of medicines which cure phlegm-fever combinations includes Tibetan quince [*bSe.yab, Chaenomeles lagenaria* (Loise)], *Iris germanica,* Coriander, Sea Buckthorn, Blue Lily, Pomegranate, Ginger and Emblic Myrobalan.

The class of medicines used to cure wind-phlegm combinations consists of (medicinal) Ginger, Ginger, Asafoetida, 'Sanchal' black salt, Onion and Garlic.

The category of medicines which cure cold phlegm conditions includes Pomegranate, Black Pepper, Longpeper, medicinal Ginger, white-flowered Leadwort, Greater Cardamon, Smaller Cardamon, Cinnamon, Indian Beech, *Embelia* (Bay breng), *Rhododendron affcephoelanthum* Franch, Black Cumin seed, *Trachyspermum amni,* (black) *Clematis, Anemone (rivularis), Ranunculus pulchellus,* white mineral salt, lake salt, rock salt, horn salt and ash salt.

Medicines used in wind disorders include Nutmeg, raw cane sugar and various bones, whilst the class of medicines for lymph disorders consists of Sal tree resin, Foetid Cassia, *Cannabis medica* and concentrate of Catechu and Indian Barberry (root).

The category of anthelmintics contains Musk, Asafoetida, Garlic, Bengal Kino tree, *Datura,* Henbane, *Embelia,* seed of *Iris ensata,* Snail shell, *Artemesia (nestita)* ash, *Daphne tangutica* (tibetanum), *Arisaema, Zanthoxylum* and *Heracleum (candicans).*

The class of anti-diarrhoeals consists of both wild and cultivated types of Bael fruit, *Schizandra sphaerandra,* Acorn, powdered root (of, for example, old pine tree), Plantain (*Plantago depressa*), *Plantago lanceolata,* Bastard Teak, the blood of Hodgson's antelope and Larkspur (*Delphinium grandiflora* Linn.)

In the category of oedema medicines are included lake salt, rock salt, golden sand, crab, Smaller Cardamon and (a type of) Mallow leaf (*Malva verticillata*).

The class of emetics contains pericarp of Soapnut, Hill Dockleaf, Thistle (*Cirsium* sp.), Sweet Flag Root, *Thladiantha harmsii* Cogn., *Fragaria nilgeerensis* (a type of mock strawberry), seed of *Sophora moorcroftiana*, *Pyrola incarnata* and mustard seed.

The category of medicines inducing purgation includes (long-tipped) Chebulic myrobalan, Castor Oil seed, Cassia pods, Euphorbia sp., Physic nut (*Baliospermum montanum*), *Euphorbia pallassii*, *Rheum emodi* (a type of rhubarb), *Lactuca dissecta* (a type of larkspur), *Physalis peruviana*, *Rheum nobile*,[1] *Stellera chamaejasme* and *chhu.rtsa* (*Rheum spiciforme*).

Methods of compounding are twofold: (a) according to taste and (b) according to power.

Compounding according to taste [gives rise to] fifty-seven combinations.

[When] two tastes are compounded there are five sweet [combinations: sweet and sour, sweet and salty, sweet and bitter, sweet and hot, and sweet and astringent]; four sour [combinations]: [sour and salty, sour and bitter, sour and hot, and sour and astringent]; three salty [combinations: salty and bitter, salty and hot, and salty and astringent]; two bitter [combinations: bitter and hot, and bitter and astringent], and a single hot [combination of hot and astringent] making a total of fifteen dual combinations.

(When) three tastes are compounded there are ten sweet [combinations]: [(1) sweet, sour and salty; (2) sweet, sour and bitter; (3) sweet, sour and hot; (4) sweet, sour and astringent; (5) sweet, salty and bitter; (6) sweet, salty and hot; (7) sweet, salty and astringent; (8) sweet, bitter and hot; (9) sweet, bitter and astringent; (10) sweet, hot and astringent]; six sour [combinations: (1) sour, salty and bitter; (2) sour, salty and hot; (3) sour, salty and astringent; (4) sour, bitter and hot; (5) sour, bitter and astringent; (6) sour, hot and astringent;] three salty [combinations: (1) salty, bitter and hot; (2) salty, bitter and astringent; (3) salty, hot and astringent]; and a single bitter [combination: bitter, hot and astringent].

(When) four [tastes] are compounded there are ten sweet [combinations: (1) sweet, sour, salty and bitter, (2) sweet, sour, salty and hot, (3) sweet, sour, salty and astringent, (4) sweet, sour, bitter and hot, (5) sweet, sour, bitter and astringent, (6) sweet, sour, hot and astringent; (7) sweet, salty, bitter and hot; (8) sweet, salty, bitter and astringent; (9) sweet, salty, hot and astringent; (10) sweet, bitter, hot and astringent]; four sour [combinations: (1) sour, salty, bitter and hot; (2) sour, salty, bitter and astringent; (3) sour, salty, hot and astringent; (4) sour, bitter, hot and astringent]; and a single salty [combination: salty, bitter, hot and astringent].

When five (tastes) are compounded there are five sweet [combinations: (1) sweet, sour, salty, bitter and hot; (2) sweet, sour, salty, bitter and astringent; (3) sweet, sour, bitter, hot and astringent; (4) sweet, sour, salty, hot and astringent; (5) sweet, salty, bitter, hot and astringent] and a single sour [combination: sour, salty, bitter, hot and astringent].

[Therefore] there are fifteen [combinations] of four tastes and [fifteen] of two tastes, six [combinations] of five tastes, twenty [combinations] of three tastes and a single six-[taste] compound. [These together with the] six single tastes [make a total of] sixty-three. Remedies for the seventy-four increases and decreases [of the humors] are to be compounded [accordingly].

Compounding according to power is twofold: pacification and purging.

The compounding of pacification medicines has five or seven sections. The five are: (a) decoction, (b) powder, (c) pill, (d) extract, (e) medicinal oils (which, with the addition of) both (f) medicinal wine and (g) desiccated syrup (including concentrates), may be enumerated as seven.

Purging includes suppositories, purgatives, emetics, enemas and nasal cleansing (therapy). These remove [disorders involving collective imbalances of] all three humors and headaches [arising therefrom].

The remedies for the four hundred and four diseases thus have been enumerated. This concludes the twenty-first chapter from *The Quintessence Tantra, the Secret Oral Tradition of the Eight Branches of the Science of Healing*.

22. Medical Instruments

Then the sage Yid.las.skyes asked: O Master, Sage Rig.pahi.ye.she, how may one learn the principles of instruments and (accessory) therapy? May the Healer, King of Physicians, please explain.

Having been thus requested the Teacher replied: O great sage, listen. The study of the principles of instruments and (accessory) therapy, which are the remedies for healing disease, is twofold: the therapy and the instrument used to perform it.

The actual therapy extracts disease from the outside or (serves to) subdue [the disorder] and is threefold: mild, coarse and forceful. Mild therapy in turn is threefold: fomentation, medicinal bath or embrocation, and oil massage. Coarse therapy is (also) threefold: venesection, moxabustion and (minor) surgery. Forceful therapy is fourfold: amputation, [general] surgery, extraction and expulsion.

The use of instruments includes examination of pain points to ascertain whether projectiles are lodged in the body, (the use of) forceps, scalpels, surgical spoon and minor instruments.

Forceps are used to examine for projectiles (as above). The first of these is round with a base no different from the tip and is six fingerbreadths (long). It is called *khab.mgo* (lit. 'needle head', i.e., trephine), and is used to examine for skull fractures.

The *mgo.zlum* (lit. 'roundhead'), *bra.wo* (lit.'buckwheat'), *rtse.kyog* (lit. 'curved point'), *rtse.gug* (lit. 'bent point'), *sbrul.mig* (lit. 'snake eye') and *zangs.dung.kha.hdra* (lit. 'like the mouth of a copper trumpet') are all hollow, thin, smooth and twelve fingerbreadths in length. These are used (in turn) to examine pain points in the limbs (for projectiles).

The *dpal.ldan.rtse* (lit. 'the magnificent point') is eight fingerbreadths in length, has a small hole and is used to examine whether swellings have suppurated or not.

The *shubs.chan* (lit. 'the hollow one') is three fingerbreadths in length and shaped like a cow's teat. It should be five fingerbreadths in circumference for (use on) men and six fingerbreadths long for (use on) women. To locate the diseased part, [for example hemorrhoid or pustule,] the type with two holes is used. Then, for the actual [removal], one should use such instruments as the single-holed *glo.dkar* to locate the hemorrhoid [through the hole] and (proceed to) cut it (with the inserted blade).

The category of forceps and tongs used for extracting projectiles includes *seng.ge.kha* (lit. 'lion's mouth'), *kang.ka.mchhu* (lit. 'beak of kang-ka bird') and *bya.rog.mchhu* (lit. 'crow's beak'). These are eighteen fingerbreadths in length and the cross-pieces are firmly joined at the center by a nail. The end (of the handle) is shaped like an iron hook, with a ring attached to it. These are used to extract projectiles lodged in the bone.

Similarly the eight-fingerbreadths-long *mthing.ril.mchhu* (lit. 'wild duck's beak')-like [forceps] are extremely fine for removing projectiles from the flesh and ligaments.

The hollow (probe) is twelve fingerbreadths in length, hard with a hole at the tip and containing (a thin rod). It is known as *hdam.bu.mchhu* and is used to remove projectiles from deep wounds. Also it has a thin blade and a ring attached to the handle.

tsu.ma.ti (is used to) remove necrosed (parts of) channels and ligaments.

(Those instruments) classed as lancets are indicated for removing flesh and extracting blood. They are six fingerbreadths long and resemble the hollow (center-) tube of a sparrow's feather. They are applied to the single vein inside the (layers of) flesh.

The *stag.nyal* instrument has a sharp point (used for) (extracting blood) from the *snod.ka* and *rtse.chung* veins. The axe-like blade is used to extract blood from veins above bones. The *chhu.gri* (lit. 'water knife' (used) for gutting fish)-like instrument is used to pare off swellings. The sickle-shaped instrument (*zor.wahi.dbyids*), eight fingerbreadths in length, (is used to) cut away swellings on the tongue. The lancet-like *brang.wa.chan* instrument (is used to) make incisions on the skull.

Instruments used in spoon surgery for piercing (the flesh, for example) are six fingerbreadths in length. The head (of the spoon should be wide enough to) leave room for the handle (to follow it) and the base should be heavy.

The *sbubs.thur.sbal.mgo* (lit. 'hollow frog's head') spoon clears out pockets of vapor and drains fluid (accumulations) from the heart and liver through its opening. The *sbubs.thur.myu.gu.kha* (lit. 'hollow pen mouth') spoon drains oedema fluid, whilst the *byid.pohi.mchhu.hdra* (lit. '*byid.po* bird's beak-like') spoon extracts pus (accumulations) in the trunk of the body.

The spoon with head similar to a barley (grain) is used (to remove) spinal tumors. (To remove tumors of) the lungs, heart, large and small intestines and kidneys the *sbal.mgo* (frog's head) spoon is recommended.

The copper spoon with buckwheat-like (point) disperses cataracts, etc., whilst the fifteen-centimeter-long *hbri.lche* (she-yak tongue) [spoon] is used to extract all trace (of tumors).

The blade of the *mdung.rtse* (lit. 'spear head') instrument (is used to) extract pus and fluid (accumulations) in the limbs.

Furthermore the category of minor instruments is set out (as follows):

The two *ste.kha* blades, the *be.le.kha* and *rko.mahi.mchhu* (lit. 'beak of ko-ma bird')-like blades are (each) six fingerbreadths in length and are of finely tempered metal with (wooden) handles. (These are used) to remove bone from (fractured) skulls.

The surgical saw is two fingerbreadths wide and exactly ten fingerbreadths in length (and is used) to pare away superfluous (fractured) bone. The *chhan.pa* (lit. 'scissors') is (extremely) sharp and cuts away veins and ligaments from wounds. The

hollow saw-edged blade is five fingerbreadths long, bears a
ring and makes holes in bone.

The ten-fingerbreadths-long *be.le.kha*-like instrument with
curved point (is used to) remove pustules of the ear, nose and
throat. The *mngal.thur* (lit. 'womb spoon') is fifteen centimeters
long with a curved point and (is used to) remove a dead fetus
from the womb.

The *sbrul.mgo* ('snake's head') instrument removes stones
(from the urinary bladder, etc.), whilst the *hphrul.thur* (lit.
'separating spoon') is twelve fingerbreadths long, the size of a
medium wheatstalk, hard and smooth, with a hole (at the end).
It relieves urinary retention.

The ten-fingerbreadths-long *rtse.kyog* (lit. 'curved point')
burns dental caries. The ten-fingerbreadths-long (instrument)
has a five-finger opening and two tubes through which smoke
is inhaled.

The hollow *them.bu.lta.buhi.kha* instrument is ten
fingerbreadths long and (is used to) place medicine in the
throat and to apply moxabustion to the uvula.

The instrument called *gche-hu* (Clyster pipe) is hollow at the
end to a distance of one thumb (-length), with a chickpea sized
hole at the tip and is eight fingerbreadths long. It is bound by
a ring half-way along and (is used to) apply suppository and
enema. A similar, more slender, version (of this instrument) is
used for cleaning wounds.

The *rngabs.rva* (oxhorn) instrument is five fingerbreadths
high and three fingerbreadths in diameter. It has a mustard-
seed-sized hole at the tip (through which) lymph fluid is
extracted.

The vase (*bum.pa*) (-instrument) is eighteen fingerbreadths
in circumference, twelve fingerbreadths high and (with a round
mouth some four fingerbreadths in area). It is used to disperse
and extract external tumors [and pain resulting from reactions
between blood and wind].

The standard razor resembles the (crescent of the waxing
moon) and is used for shaving the head.

The *tel.pa* instrument is ten fingerbreadths long, has a
spatula-like head and is used to cauterize abscesses, ulcers and
swellings.

The thin, smooth, (dagger)-pointed 'flesh needle' is used to stitch lacerations of the flesh and skin.

Thus such instruments are to be applied (according to the type of) disease and the requirements (at the time).

This concludes the twenty-second chapter, on instruments, from *The Quintessence Tantra, the Secret Oral Tradition of the Eight Branches of the Science of Healing.*

23. Normal health

Then sage Yid.las.skyes asked, O Great Sage Rig.pahi.ye.she, how may one learn the principles of normal (good) health? May the Healer, King of Physicians, please explain.

Having been thus requested the Teacher replied, O Great Sage, listen. The [two] unchanging aspects of the normal body are remaining free of disease and enjoying long life.

Firstly with regard to remaining healthy [one should understand that] all diseases arise from causes and conditions and it is impossible for fruition to occur from cause without [the addition of ripening] conditions. Therefore one should abandon all (ripening) conditions for disease.

With regard to season, sense organs, behavior, tastes and powers, if one indulges (these) insufficiently, to excess or in a wrong way, disease will ensue. However, perfect adjustment (to these factors) is the cause of remaining healthy. Therefore by partaking perfectly of behavioral pattern, food and medicine one will remain contented and free of disease. With the passing of years and months the strength of the bodily constituents declines, the lifespan dwindles and the afflictions of old age are lingering. (Therefore) *rejuvenation* is fourfold: (a) benefits, (b) environment, (c) working basis and (d) mode of practice.

The benefits are to provide the middle-aged with long life and youthfulness, to develop the vital energy of the body and to sharpen the sense faculties.

The environment should be clean, quiet, pleasant and free of interferences.

The working basis should not be an extremely aged person, but one who forsakes sexual desires and with persevering (mind) aligns his actions to the timely [conjunctions] of favorable planets and stars.

The mode of practice is twofold: (1) those who principally adopt [rejuvenation] and (2) those whose practice is inconsistent.

For those principally engaged there are *(a)* the preliminaries and *(b)* the actual process.

The preliminaries [commence with] the oil therapy (see chapter thirteen of the Final Tantra), followed by a bath. Then administer the [purgative] compound of the three (myrobalan) fruits, rock salt, longpeper, wild ginger, Sweet Flag, turmeric, Embelia, raw cane sugar and cow's urine as an abdominal cleanser. [Attempting rejuvenation] without such cleansing would be fruitless, like dyeing a stained cloth.

The actual process [begins with] the preparation of [the medicinal butter of] garlic and clarified butter, [which should be kept in a] container inside a heap of barley for three weeks and then taken (for the same) number of days. It cures wind disorders and promotes longevity.

[Secondly,] well-purified mineral exudate [should be added to calcinated gold, silver, copper and iron, kept in an iron container and taken] with (other) wholesome medicines. [The amount taken] should be increased in stages. [The mixture] dispels [all types of] disease and promotes longevity. However, one should abstain from taking Mon Chenopodium (*mon.sne*, the dark red 'New Year' flower) and Chinese peas (slightly flat white or brown pea).

[Thirdly,] taking a combination of Leadwort, butter and honey promotes longevity, fortifies the constitution and raises (digestive) heat.

[Fourthly,] taking (Leadwort) combined with cow's urine cures leucoderma and leprosy.

[Fifthly,] the medicinal butter of the three (myrobalan) fruits clears the sense organs, increases strength and rejuvenates.

In all cases one should apply wholesome diet and behavioral pattern to whatever disorder (prevails) and avoid rotten, sour, unwholesome foods and green leafy vegetables. The [best] results of [rejuvenation] are achieved by three, six or twelve months' [treatment], failing which, if one can undergo [only] incomplete [rejuvenation], then one will be able to gain only short-lived results.

This concludes the twenty-third chapter, on normal health, from *The Quintessence Tantra, the Secret Oral Tradition of the Eight Branches of the Science of Healing.*

24. Diagnosis

Then the sage Yid.las.skyes asked: O Great Sage Rig.pahi.ye.she, how may one learn the diagnosis (of symptoms)? May the Healer, King of Physicians, please explain.

Having been thus requested the Teacher replied: O great sage, listen. The study of the diagnosis of symptoms is like fire and the smoke (produced from it). Thus one can identify the disease by examining its symptoms. A doctor who lacks diagnostic techniques is unable to recognize symptoms as such and is like one who mistakes steam for smoke. He follows uncertain indications like one who says that rain will be produced whenever clouds gather. Therefore the techniques of diagnosis and examination are expounded (as follows).

[Firstly] examination to show the actual humor [-al nature of disease], because of a need to cure (by) divining the cause, symptoms and beneficial and harmful factors.

[Secondly,] equivocal examination [where necessary] so as to maintain the patient's morale and so that he or she will still express (faith) in the doctor's skill (chapter twenty-five).

[Thirdly,] when (faced with) curing [a patient], in order (to know whether) to accept or refuse (a patient), there are four conditions of accepting or declining (to accept) the patient (chapter twenty-six).

EXAMINATION

Examination which reveals the actual humor(-al imbalance) [is threefold]: (a) [Thorough] examination of the cause or arisal (of disease), (b) [Thorough] examination of symptoms and (c) [Thorough] examination assessing (factors which have proved) beneficial or harmful.

With regard to diet and behavior (which act as) causes and conditions for the arisal [of disease] one may understand all ailments [by questioning about the patient's recent] diet and activities. In particular the [immediate] conditions of arisal will be recognized, for how could dissimilar fruit possibly be produced from (any one type of) cause?

Recognizing symptoms has four aspects: (a) the basis of examination, (b) the objects of examination, (c) the doors of examination and (d) the methods of examination.

The basis of examination consists of wind, bile and phlegm, the symptoms of which are diagnosed according to their increase, decrease, accumulation, arisal and disruption. Also one should examine whether (these are) to be subsumed under hot or cold (types of disorder).

The objects of examination (consist of) the five sense organs and their objects as well as the five impurities. The sense organs comprise the eye, ear, nose, tongue and body (that feels), and their five objects are form, sound, smell, taste and objects of touch. Examination may also be made of the five excretions: mucus, loose motions, vomit, urine and blood.

In order to diagnose without error one should check (all) *the doors [of examination]*, namely the environment, the season, the (humoral) nature (of the patient), his or her age, the time of day, intake of food and seat (of disease).

Methods of examination involve visual examination, feeling (for example, the pulse) and questioning.

The objects of the doctor's visual examination are the size, shape and color (of the body), and in particular one should check the tongue and urine. Such is the discriminating examination of visual objects.

Diagnosis by feeling entails examining whether areas of the body are hot, cold, smooth or uneven. In particular one should examine the pulse, which is (like) a messenger who bears news and which is to be analyzed and its significance examined with discrimination.

Examination by questioning includes all objects of audial [consciousness]. One should examine the (immediate) causes, symptoms, seat (of disease) and environmental factors, and in particular enquire about the causes, location and symptoms. From the causes one [ascertains] the humor[-al nature of the disorder], (whilst) from the location one recognizes the entrances (of the disease) and from the symptoms one distinguishes the specific types of disease. Thus questioning is essential in all examinations, according to the art of [analyzing] sounds as explained (above).

Depending on what is harmful or beneficial one should rely on the fourfold food, behavioral pattern, medicine and accessory therapy. (Moreover) one should (check) whether the causes and nature of the disease correspond or not and all disorders will be identified [without error by analyzing] wholesome and unwholesome factors. Rather than rely on [superficial] appearance, thorough examination should be conducted, for once the doctor has realized the state (of the disorder) he will [easily] discern the required treatment.

This concludes the twenty-fourth chapter, on diagnosis, from *The Quintessence Tantra, the Secret Oral Tradition of the Eight Branches of the Science of Healing.*

25. Examination by Craft and Guile

Then Sage Rig.pahi.ye.she spoke these words: O Great Sage, listen. Examination by craft and guile (has eight aspects): (1) recognizing symptoms, (2) detecting faults, (3) to take one's time, (4) previous treatment, (5) 'putting the patient on the spot', (6) 'cutting the patient short', (7) 'reaching one's peak' and (8) 'ducking the issue'.

Firstly with regard to *recognizing symptoms*, one should diagnose all disorders (on) a general and specific basis. Merely by having recognized this much one will be able to (fore)see the development of the disorder. Therefore it is essential to have a comprehensive and intimate knowledge of diagnostic principles. (For example), although one may recognize precious gems, etc., as being of fine or poor [quality], [conclusive examination] is not possible without a text [describing their individual features] or if one has no training in how to do this.

Detecting faults [refers to] the method of relating to the messenger whereby one gains a clear understanding of which [part of the patient's body is affected], the [external] symptoms, what [food and medicines] have been given, who [his doctor is] and how many days [have passed since the onset of disease]. (These aspects) are analyzed without having spoken [directly to the patient].

Taking one's time entails remaining (at ease) for the moment in an unhurried manner. [The doctor] should undistractedly analyze [on the basis of the patient's] account and actions of body, speech and mind.

(With regard to) *previous treatment* one should investigate what was done [in the way] of venesection, moxabustion and medication. Merely through having found out this one will gain an adequate understanding [of the patient's disorder in terms of] hot and cold.

[With regard to] '*putting the patient on the spot*': establishing the essence, if [the patient] says nothing at all [to indicate his symptoms] and if one does not understand [the nature of his condition], one should not intimidate him to (make him) divulge [his symptoms]. [Rather the doctor should say, "First] I need to remedy the spirit disorder [troubling you and then] I'll prepare a medicine which may help you". Because of such a non-committal pronouncement the patient cannot accept [what is proposed, because he worries that the disease might be fatal since the doctor has not promised a cure, and so] in this way is led to reveal whatever [the doctor needs to know].

In the case of what is known as '*cutting the patient short*', the doctor encounters a certain patient who describes [most of his symptoms]. Once one has gained an understanding from such an account (one can say), "The doctor understands whatever [is wrong with you] and does not need your explanation". Then, because of one's recounting (also the remaining) symptoms people will say one is a remarkable physician.

With regard to the techniques known as '*reaching one's peak*', if one has [unmistakenly] diagnosed [the disorder] using the techniques [mentioned above] one can say, "Other (doctors) need to examine by pulse, urine and many other methods. I am not like them, for I am concerned with divining [the nature of disease by using only] one of these." [The patient will think, "For this doctor] mere looking is enough [to diagnose disease]", and one's renown will grow. Otherwise, because of one's thorough analysis of the patient's condition, one will be acclaimed as an expert in diagnostic (techniques).

'*Ducking the issue*': when all [the above methods have revealed no] information [regarding symptoms, etc., one's response should take] the form of divining and then one should 'play safe'. In the first case (one should say), "[Your disorder is] caused by unwholesome diet and conduct and by spirits. (In particular) you have been affected by rather sour, raw [food] and extreme exertion." (Therefore) one should prescribe a balanced remedy (placebo) which is neither beneficial nor harmful.

With regard to '*playing safe*' one should give both the disorder and the medicine names which are hitherto unheard-of, understood by no-one but (nonetheless) strikingly plausible. Thus, although by such methods he has not come to diagnose (the disorder) still [the doctor] will be acclaimed as having exceptional skill.

This concludes the twenty-fifth chapter, on examination by craft and guile, from *The Quintessence Tantra, the Secret Oral Tradition of the Eight Branches of the Science of Healing*.

26. Four Diagnostic Criteria for Accepting or Declining to Accept a Patient

Then Sage Rig.pahi.ye.she spoke these words: O Great Sage, listen. There are four diagnostic criteria for accepting or declining to accept [a patient] according to whether he or she is (1) easy, or (2) difficult to cure, (3) barely treatable, or (4) to be refrained from accepting.

(1) *The patient is easy to cure* (a) if the essential conditions are present, (b) if factors related to the patient facilitate a cure, and (c) if he or she is readily curable by virtue of [the nature of] the disease.

(a) The cure is facilitated by the three factors of a doctor, medicine and nurse (being present). The doctor should have reached the pinnacle of his or her knowledge and should be well-versed in the meaning of the texts. He or she should be [well-trained in] observation [of the practice of his or her own teacher] and [should be endowed with faultless, compassionate,] pure [mind].

The medicines are to be compounded according to (standard) methods, according to their manifold secondary qualities, their being in perfect condition and their harmonious [tastes, powers, elements, etc.]

The nurse should be efficient, caring, pure [in body, speech and mind] and intelligent [in following the doctor's instructions.] These are the twelve factors which facilitate a cure.

(b)   The patient should be a young man of controlled manner who has courage and who has good physical tolerance of all medicines. He should be affluent, capable of heeding [the doctor's] instructions and able to understand [the causes and conditions of disease]. (Finally) if he is proficient at describing his symptoms when asked then he will be easy to cure.[1]

(c)   Readily curable by virtue of [the nature of] the disease: If the causes of disease, the prior means (of arisal) and the external signs (and symptoms) are slight, and if the affected part [e.g., bodily constituent], the location, season and (humoral) nature do not match, [the patient will be easy to cure]: (e.g., if one contracts a bile disorder in a wind-location such as in the bones or in any cold-natured location or in a cool season such as a monsoon, it will be easy to cure). [Similarly if the patient's condition is] unaffected [by any additional or secondary disorder, if the disorder follows only] one path it is a single humoral imbalance or if of fresh onset then a cure will be easily effected. Moreover in the case of a contagious fever occurring in a matching (hot) location and season or in dysuria (urinary retention or anuria) counterbalanced [by stool or urine] in the affected area or in the case of a chronic blood tumor a cure will also be easily effected.

(2)   In cases which are difficult to treat the 'easy' syndromes [above are complicated] by being mixed (with other factors), or the disorder requires a great deal of treatment over a prolonged period.

(3)   In contrast (to (1) and (2) above) *one who is barely treatable* [will not benefit from medication and his condition will only] respond to [the diet and behavioral pattern with which he was previously] familiar. Thus he may live out the remainder of his life.

(4)   The type of patient one should refrain from accepting is

twofold according to whether (a) a means of administering treatment exists or (b) not.

(a)   If the patient bears animosity towards the King,
spiritual master or living beings, lacks gratitude
for the doctor's past efforts, disparages the doctor, lacks [the time to take treatment], is not a man
of means, cannot obey [instructions], if his lifespan
is exhausted, if he is overcome by sorrow,
destroys the Holy Doctrine [of the Lord Buddha]
or if others ascribe to him a bad reputation, it is
therefore stated that (the doctor) should decline
to accept him even if a means of administering
treatment exists [because the above factors will
adversely affect the doctor].

(b)   With respect to the type of patient who is not to
be accepted in view of the absence of a means of
treatment, if he is beyond hope, bears the signs
of death, or if he is seized by (any of) the nine fatal
diseases [the doctor] should not accept him.

This was the twenty-sixth chapter, on four diagnostic criteria
for accepting or declining to accept [a patient], from *The
Quintessence Tantra, the Secret Oral Tradition of the Eight
Branches of the Science of Healing.*

27. Principles of Therapeutics

Then the Sage Yid.las.skyes asked: O Master, Sage Rig.pahi.ye.she, how may one learn the principles of therapeutics? May the Healer, King of Physicians, please explain.

At this the Master said: O Great Sage, listen. Once the disorder has been diagnosed, in order to treat it I shall present the principles of therapeutics. [These are twofold:] (1) therapeutic techniques and (2) remedial measures. First I shall present the therapeutic procedures. Although there are indeed countless remedial measures, using them without therapeutic techniques is like shooting arrows in the dark.

THERAPEUTIC TECHNIQUES

This [section is threefold:] (a) general, (b) individual and (c) specific therapeutic techniques.

General Therapeutic Techniques

The first of these is presented in three parts: (1) the method of healing, (2) the remedy which heals and (3) extent of treatment.

(1) The method of healing. Firstly any (type of) disorder of wind, etc., should be eliminated at its own location in the season of its accumulation. If this is not done then [in the monsoon when the wind disorder] has arisen and has grown

(strong) it therefore creates the disturbance of other [humoral] disorders. One should then treat (e.g.,) by compounds, suppositories or pacification which do not disturb other [humors]. [If, however,] other [humoral] disorders are produced then the most pronounced disorder is to be treated (first) followed by treatment for the other secondary humoral imbalances.

(2) The remedy which heals is twofold: (a) pacification [medicines] and (b) [evacuation]. In the season of accumulation [of wind] one should pacify [the disorder], whereas once it has arisen [e.g., in monsoon] one should treat by means of evacuation.

At the time of pacification (e.g., of wind) one should be careful with respect to diet and behavioral pattern so as not to disturb [the other humors]. However, when the (corresponding) circumstances and conditions (are present) out of season then the accumulation and arisal of (humoral) disorders [will occur at such times]. Because it is difficult to treat [a humoral disorder] once its season is past one should cure it promptly [by means of medication]. The medicine should be administered over twenty-four hours according to mealtimes, and discriminatingly applied according to the disorder (i.e., at times when the humoral imbalance is at its peak. There are also said to be ten methods of administering it. The medication should be administered) (1) when the stomach is empty (early in the morning), (2) just before the meal, (3) half way through the meal, (4) just after the meal, (5) between mouthfuls of food, (6) immediately following digestion, (7) at no (specific) time, i.e., repeatedly in small doses as required, e.g., in the case of asthma, (8) mixed with food [as in the case of anorexia,] (9) just before and just after a meal [as in the case of hiccoughs,] or (10) at night upon retiring [when the evening meal has already been digested, e.g., for disorders occurring above the level of the throat]. Administering medicine for all (disorders) at times not corresponding [to the humoral imbalance] and (only) when digestion has taken place is a foolish system, and it will then be difficult to strike at the heart of the disorder. [Thus the administration of medication at the appropriate times] is like being able to distinguish between [white and black] pebbles.

(3) Extent of treatment. Whenever treatment is applied to any disorder and much sputum or mucus appear with heavi-

ness of the body, anorexia, indigestion, drying up of the flow [of the bodily constituents or excretions] or decomposing [of the excretions], irregular passing of stool and urine, debility and vocal weakness, these are signs that (either) the disorder is not being cured at all [or that it is not being collected for the treatment to be able to dispel it]. Whenever any disorder is pacified, opposite signs to the above appear.

[Until the disorder is pacified one should firmly persevere with] the treatment and once it is pacified superfluous treatment should not be applied.

Individual Therapeutic Techniques

Individual therapeutic techniques are threefold: (1) [any disorder] accompanied by indigestion, (2) single humoral imbalances, (3) other-powered disorders [i.e., bi- or tri-humoral disorders].

(1) Disorders accompanied by indigestion. In the first case when the digestive heat is low then food and drink [and nutriment] will not be digested. Then this indigestion together with a [humoral imbalance] of wind, etc. becomes mixed with the objects of harm [i.e., with the seven bodily constituents and the three excretions.]. (One should therefore) administer medicine to ripen the disorder or to increase the digestive heat and thereby reduce the disorder. When the signs of such having been accomplished are achieved one should evacuate the disorder through its nearest location [i.e., by emesis if localized in the upper body and by purgation if localized in the lower body].

If of its own accord vomiting or purging occurs one should not block these processes with medication. Until the disorder has ripened one should not apply evacuation because to do so would cause the imbalanced humor(s) to mingle with the bodily constituents and impair them. [This can be compared to the example of straining off the liquid from grain beer before it has fermented (and thus ruining the grain)].

(2) Single humoral imbalances. With respect to single humoral disorders unaccompanied by indigestion the cause for all disorders to be generated is the initial onset of a wind imbalance caused by unsuitable dietary and behavioral factors followed by the onset of other disorders. If the dietary and

behavioral [conditions] are not assembled in the season [when the single humoral disorder would naturally] arise then the disorder will accumulate in its own (natural) location, abide for a long time and not gain the power [to manifest]. For example, it is like a conflict between opponents; [the weaker one] will not retaliate [until he has found support from others]. (Similarly) when the (precipitating) conditions are met with and (the disorder) has gained power then it will arise from its location. Prior to [the onset of other disorders] a wind disorder will occur because of which the other humors will be disturbed. When [appropriate dietary and behavioral factors] have reduced the wind disorder the digestive bile therefore [increases in power], and when it has ripened [the formerly unripened disorder], the latter is then scattered by the wind. [This wind] should be halted so that the disorder can be collected internally. For example, it is similar to abating a wind to permit rain to fall.

Next one should evacuate [the disorder by purgation or emesis] through whichever pathway is nearer. If one is not [able to] collect internally [the disorder] from the limbs and outer locations [where it has been scattered] one should externally [perform venesection] at the openings of the veins and also cleanse them from within.

(3) Other-powered disorders. An other-powered [disorder] is a [humoral] disorder accompanied by a secondary disorder. E.g., when [bile] rises from its [natural] location (by force of wind) and enters another [e.g., wind] location, from there it [returns] to its own former location to harm and disturb [the wind abiding there]. Once the power [of the wind] diminishes, one should treat [the bile disorder] in its own former location. [If, however, the wind] later increases in power, then by treating this secondary disorder the primary bile disorder abiding in its own (natural) location will be cured without requiring treatment. This is similar to a master who relies upon a servant (or accomplice) to commit a burglary. (If one overcomes the prime conspirator it is easy to prevail over the accomplice).

Specific Therapeutic Techniques
    Specific therapeutic techniques have nine aspects:
    (1) If one fails to realize [the nature of the disorder] and feels doubtful, then one should experimentally treat the

unascertained disorder in the way that a cat lies in wait [for a mouse: if one suspects a wind disorder, one should just administer wind medicine in small doses and then change the treatment if the condition does not respond.]

(2) When one has identified [the disorder], ascertained its nature and become convinced thereof one should treat [the disorder] in a direct manner [which may be] likened to hoisting a flag on a mountain top.

(3) If the remedial measures do not strike at [the disorder] then one should follow its pathway and treat in the manner of training a wild horse to run a race. [According to the reason for the medication not performing its function one should either ripen or collect or separate the elements of the disorder.]

(4) Having examined why previous treatment of [the patient's] disorder was inadequate, excessive or erroneous, one should treat it in the manner of a kingfisher catching fish [i.e., in a precise, direct manner after ascertaining which of the above three] faults affected the previous treatment.

(5) In the case of a serious disorder one should apply dietary and behavioral factors, medication and accessory therapies, i.e., treat with powerful remedial measures in the manner of someone who strikes [first to eliminate] his enemy when he encounters him in a narrow impasse.

(6) If the disorder is mild then one should gradually apply behavioral and dietary factors, medication and accessory therapy each in turn, i.e., treat in the manner of one who climbs a staircase step by step.

(7) In the case of a single humoral disorder, just as a hero [directly and unmistakenly] subdues his adversary, one should treat with compounds which do not harm the other humors.

(8) In disorders (involving) dual or triple humoral imbalances one should treat in a balanced way, i.e., in the manner of an arbiter who resolves a dispute between opponents.

(9) In all such cases, to the objects of harm ten factors should be applied and treatment should be according to the level (of the disorder), i.e., like the load of a Dzo or the load of a sheep [these two should not be exchanged. In the same way mild medicine should be administered for a mild disorder and powerful medication for a serious one].

Thus it was said.

This concludes the twenty-seventh chapter, expounding general therapeutics, from *The Quintessence Tantra, the Secret Oral Tradition of the Eight Branches of the Science of Healing.*

28. Specific Therapeutic Techniques

Then the Sage Yid.las.skyes asked: O Master, Sage Rig.pahi.ye.she.la, specific therapeutic techniques were taught in brief as having nine aspects. What is the detailed extensive (exposition) of these? Thus it was said.

The Master replied: O Great Sage, listen. With respect to the detailed exposition of therapeutic techniques, *(1)* in the first instance, *if one is in doubt* when one analyses the symptoms of a disorder then e.g., (a) in the case of a wind disorder one should (administer) the soup of sheep's ankle bone as a probe; (b) in the case of a bile disorder one should use Chiretta decoction as a probe, whilst (c) in a phlegm disorder one should apply the threefold rock salt [decoction]. (d) As a probe for infections or parasitic disorders or for disorders of the stomach and large intestine one should use the Garuda five compound. (e) As a probe in disturbed blood disorders and wind-pain (neuralgia) the fourfold *Iris germanica* decoction is applied. (f) In the case [of disorders] caused by compounded poisons, as a probe one should administer a collecting compound [e.g., thirteenfold collector decoction]. (g) In mixed hot and cold disorders, as a probe one should rely upon one's experience [e.g., the dietary and behavioral factors with which one is familiar.] (h) To check the advisability of using a laxative one should administer the *sna.sel.khrog* ('slight rumbling') decoction. (i) As a probe [to confirm whether it is appropriate] to apply moxabustion one should apply a hot oil fomentation, (j) and as a (similar) probe for venesection one should apply either a cold stone or sprinkle [cool] water. (k) To test for pus one should pierce with the hollow-fire-spoon (surgical instrument). In the case of other disorders with regard to which one has suspicions [or doubts] as a probe one should resort to (giving) small quantities of (the appropriate) remedial compounds. In all cases of mixed and facsimiles of dual (humoral) disorders one should compare [the disorder] by administering whatever remedy [is appropriate since] it is of prime importance to treat (the disorder). One should be circumspect rather than explicit [whilst still endeavoring to ascertain the nature of the disorder]. At such times one should speak in veiled terms rather than make clear pronouncements.

(2) Once one has ascertained and become convinced of [the nature of] the disorder [one can state] which causes and conditions have produced it and then what [nature and location the disorder] will adopt in its final stages. [The physician can then affirm] how the disorder should be treated and what period of time will be required (to effect) a cure. However, if [a cure] is not possible one should reveal the time of death [if it is imminent]. Such speech making [the facts] known to all is likened to the flag flown on the (mountain) peak.

(3) If the remedy does not strike upon [the disorder], it will be difficult [for the former] to enter the path of (i.e., cure) [the latter]. [Cool-powered medicines given as] a remedy for unripened fever will strike upon its accomplices (i.e., wind and phlegm) and, by increasing these accomplices, increase the fever itself. Therefore those accomplices, phlegm and wind, should be separated by decoction [of *Iris germanica* no.4, etc.] Diseased blood [mixed with the pure] constitutional blood is similar to a mixture of water and milk. Therefore so as to be able to perform venesection one should separate the waste blood (by administering) the 'three (myrobalan) fruits' decoction. If one does not separate them in this way, harm to the bodily constituents will result. For example, (in the cases of) scattered [brown] phlegm and poison-fever one should collect the disorder (so as to) eradicate it. If the disorder is not collected then remedial (measures) will disperse the disorder again instead of healing it.

[In the case of] hidden fever, one should [first] remove the cold covering [layer of phlegm or wind] by means of warm [-powered medication]. This is because [otherwise] due to the cold factors the fever will not respond [favorably to cool] medication.

In all cases of indigestion one should either ripen the disorder or administer heat-inducing medicines. Once one gains the signs of having subdued the peak of the disorder one should purge it through the nearest pathway [i.e., by purgation or emesis as appropriate].

A preliminary purgative uproots all disorders, [however if one is] not [able to] uproot the disorder in this way, then it is like water falling upon ice (i.e., just as the ice will not be melted so the disorder will not be dispelled.)

(4) [Like a kingfisher]. When [a patient] has been previously treated by another physician and if his disorder [has not responded to the treatment] because of inadequately or excessively (strong) or wrong (medication), one should thoroughly examine [why no recovery has come about]. If the disorder has not been pacified due to inadequate [treatment] one should administer [a stronger] remedy. In the case of erroneous (treatment) causing the disorder to grow strong, one should change the compound, whereas if, because of excessively strong treatment a secondary disorder has arisen, one should dispel it [with appropriate medication.]

(5) Meeting the enemy in a narrow impasse. (a) In the case of disorders involving a high fever one should apply the 'four waters'[1]. Camphor and venesection at the 'small point' vein are (respectively) the 'waters' of medication and accessory therapy. Fasting is the dietary 'water' and remaining in a cool place is the treatment by means of behavioral factors. (b) In the case of a [strongly] cold-powered disorder one should 'ignite the four fires': the fire of medication is a compound of all types of heat-inducing (ingredients) whilst the fire of accessory therapy is moxabustion. Warm-powered, nutritious (foods) are the dietary fire, whereas remaining in a warm place and wearing warm clothing constitute treatment by the fire of behavioral factors. If treatment is not applied in this way, then the disorder will increase endangering the life (of the patient).

(6) Rung by rung up a ladder. In mild disorders one should

214   *Quintessence Tantras of Tibetan Medicine*

first cautiously (resort to) behavioral factors. If the [disorder] is not alleviated thereby (one should) determine which foods are beneficial and which are harmful [and administer accordingly]. If these fail to alleviate the condition [one should check, whether] cool-powered or warm-powered medication is beneficial and treat (accordingly).

In case these three methods fail to eradicate the disorder one should expel it from its location by means of accessory therapy.

(7) Like the hero overcoming the enemy. In the case of all single humoral disorders of wind, bile or phlegm, when alleviating such, one should treat without producing any other (secondary) disorder. If one fails to understand this, then [any of] the twelve reaction imbalances may occur. When wrong [treatment] fails to alleviate (the disorder) itself then a secondary disorder will be created; e.g., in a wind disorder, if one relies upon bitter and hot-tasting [diet and medicines] the wind will not be alleviated, and reaction imbalances of phlegm and bile [will result from the bitter and hot tastes respectively]. If one relies upon salty and hot [-tasting diet and medicine] in a bile disorder the latter will not be alleviated, and both phlegm and wind reaction imbalances [will result from the two tastes respectively]. Bitter and salty [-tasting diet and medicines] administered in a [phlegm] disorder will fail to alleviate the phlegm and [respectively produce] reaction imbalances of both wind and bile. By [a combination of such] unwholesome conditions triple humoral reaction imbalance [will be produced], whereas by excessively [strong diet and medication a disorder will be alleviated but not without] giving rise to a further secondary condition: e.g., (extremely) sweet and salty [medicine, etc.] will alleviate wind and (respectively) produce imbalance(s) of phlegm and bile. (Moreover) hot [-tasting] and sour [medication, etc.] will alleviate phlegm and (respectively) increase wind and bile. Sweet and bitter [compounds, etc.] alleviate bile and then [respectively] produce [imbalances] of phlegm and wind.

(8) In dual and triple (humoral) disorders [one should administer] a balanced [medicine having both warm and cool powers] in combination, e.g., Myrobalan and mineral exudate generally have a balanced (remedial effect) on combined (humoral disorders). In such cases the [recommended] individual

supplementary ingredients should be added according to the location and fundamental [humoral, etc. nature] of the disorder. [The recommended additives in each case are as follows:] nutmeg is to be administered for heart conditions, bamboo concretion for the lungs, saffron for the liver, clove for the 'life-channel' (life-meridian), smaller cardamon for the kidneys, greater cardamon for the spleen, and pomegranate and longpeper for the stomach. One should add Chiretta and bitter cucumber in the case of [a secondary] bile disorder; nutmeg, Heart-leaved moonseed and soup of the three [types of bone] for wind disorders; *Iris germanica*, coriander and *Chaenomeles tibetica* for phlegm; *Adhatoda vasica* and *Picrorhiza kurroa* for blood disorders; Sal tree resin, Foetid Cassia and *Cannabis indica* for lymph disorders; and musk and Indian Baellium resin for infections and spirit disorders.

These additives are to be compounded as required according to [the disorder] and its symptoms. [When any number of these conditions are] all combined together, all the appropriate supplementary ingredients should be administered. In cases of dual or triple combined disorders, according to whether the humors are equally [imbalanced] or whether one (or more) predominates, appropriate [supplementary ingredients] should also be added to the remedies according to [which humors] predominate. Either one should in an alternating manner treat [the previously (greater humoral imbalance) and subsequently treat (a lesser one), or remove (the disorder) at one time with the remedy directly opposing it.] (For example), bile fever should be eliminated at noon and midnight, i.e., by applying cool-powered medication and dietary factors at these times of fever. At dusk and first thing in the morning one should sustain the digestive heat and treat any cold phlegm imbalance with warm-powered medication and dietary factors. In the evening and around dawn one should cater for wind, i.e., by immediately responding to the slightest wind [imbalance with] warm-powered nutritious medication and dietary factors.

[If one humor] increases excessively, it will antagonize the remaining two humors like a son [who overrides his two brothers by force of his far greater power and affluence]. (However,) if [one humor] diminishes, it should be sustained just like a bad wife (who has become such only because of

neglect). Therefore one should eliminate increases or decreases of any of the humors and restore them to a balanced
state. The bodily constituents are like the production materials
and should not be wasted. Since the stomach is like a field one
should sustain the digestive heat. Thus if one understands
[these principles] one will become a healer-physician.

(9) *Not putting a dzo's load on a sheep* or vice versa. By
means of the ten factors of the objects of harm [the seven bodily
constituents and the three excretions], the environment, the
season [and time of day], the (humoral) nature (of the person),
his age, the natural elements of the disorder, the digestive heat,
his strength and habits, one should minutely examine the
subtlest symptoms. If these are all alike [in nature] one should
administer [appropriately] strong remedial medication. If this is
not the case (one should administer a suitably moderate
dosage).

Thus it was said.

This concludes the twenty-eighth chapter, expounding the
specific therapeutic techniques, from *The Quintessence Tantra,
the Secret Oral Tradition of the Eight Branches of the Science of
Healing.*

29. Two Therapeutic Media

Then the Sage Rig.pahi.ye.she spoke as follows: O Great Sage, listen. Although the therapeutic techniques applied by the physician are numerous, they are twofold: (1) ordinary and (2) specific (chapter thirty). With respect to the ordinary one there are (a) two objects of healing, and therefore (b) two therapeutic methods.

Two Objects of Healing
    Those who [need to] gain strength should gain weight whilst others [who are overweight] should lose weight by fasting.
    Gaining weight entails the five factors of the object (the patient), the method, the advantages, the faults of excess (use) and the therapeutic means to be employed in this latter case. With respect to the object, in the instances of someone severely affected by a wind imbalance, deficiency of the bodily constituents, exhausted newlyweds, loss of blood following childbirth, punctured lung, old age, loss of sleep, grief, asceticism, exhaustion following exertion or in the summer, invariably treatment by weight increase should be applied. This should be done by a nutritious diet of mutton, raw cane sugar, white sugar, butter, milk, curd, grain beer, etc. With respect to medication one should administer a medicinal oil suitable for the disorder. The accessory therapies of suppository, bathing and massage should be applied, whilst weight should also be

gained by means of behavioral factors such as sleep, relaxation and by keeping the mind happy. By these means strength is increased and all disorders are dispelled; for example, this is likened to the way in which one who abuses gains the power [so as to produce effects by his abuse]. Overly excessive use [of the above methods produces] obesity and thereafter sores, tumorous growths, [mental] dullness, polyuria, (throat) mucus, and increases phlegm. In such cases dietary factors and medication to reduce phlegm and fat will be beneficial; e.g., Indian Baellium (black sal tree) resin, mineral exudate and Barberry bark concentrate compounded with honey will remove all types of obesity. (Alternatively) the three (myrobalan) fruits compounded with honey or wild ginger, potash, Embelia, emblic myrobalan, and [unroasted] barley flour compounded with honey remove obesity. It is better to be thin than fat, and weight increase should be moderated.

Fasting is fivefold: (a) the object, i.e., the person who needs to lose weight; (b) [the means whereby weight is reduced;] (c) the benefits; (d) the faults of excess (application); and (e) the therapeutic means of remedying the latter.

(a) With respect to the object [to be treated:] in cases of indigestion, [of one who habitually eats oily foods,] of the "stiff-thigh" [wind disorder], infectious fever, excess urination, internal ulcers, gout, rheumatism, spleen disorders, disorders of the larynx, cerebral disorders, cardiac disorders, febrile diarrhoea, vomiting, torpor, loss of appetite, constipation, urinary retention, obesity, lymph disorders and severe combined phlegm-bile syndromes. If the patient is a strong adult, treatment should be by fasting during wintertime [for three days]. Medication for such cases is of two types: (1) pacification and (2) evacuation.

Pacification entails balancing the imbalanced [elements of wind, bile and phlegm] by treatment entailing a combination of dietary and behavioral factors, medication and accessory therapy. If the patient is weak, he should abstain from food and drink [for three days] and thereafter partake of small amounts of light, easily digestible foods. If the patient is of medium strength [he should fast] and one should prescribe decoctions, powders, etc., and whatever compounds are suitable to produce heat and ripen [the phlegm]. In the case of a strong person treatment should be by means of [the above] as well as by strenuous exercise, both night and day, as well as by accessory therapies such as sudorifics, moxabustion, fomentation, embrocation and venesection.

Evacuation (is performed by) raising the disorder and then expelling it. If the disorder is in the pre-digestive phase (i.e., in the stomach), evacuation should be by means of an emetic compound whereas if it is in the post-digestive phase one should expel it by means of an enema. If the disorder is widespread one should administer a purgative, or apply a channel cleanser in the case of a channel disorder.

Pacification and evacuation reduce strength but the benefits thereof are clarity of the sense organs, physical lightness, a healthy appetite, energy in all actions, timely hunger and thirst and smooth flow of stool and intestinal gas.

Over-application of these consumes the bodily constituents, produces emaciation; vertigo; insomnia; dullness of complexion; hoarseness; sensory debility; thirst; anorexia; pain in the calf muscle, thighs, coccyx, ribs, heart and brain; attacks of contagious fever; nausea; and wind disorders. In such cases all kinds of weight-increasing media will prove beneficial. Specifically one should eat the meat of carnivorous animals, apply suppositories, and sleep having eaten one's fill. Thus one will gain weight after the fashion of a pig. Once one has gained weight there is nothing more life-giving than meat. In short one should not do anything to weaken the strength of one who has gained weight [by the above means]. However if evacuation therapy proves necessary only a mild [laxative] should be used. If weight loss is mandatory then weight increase therapy should be avoided, but in the case of a wind increase, if either of the other humors is decreased, one should apply weight increase therapy. When wind decreases and phlegm or bile increase, the patient should fast. The mode of treatment is the same when any bodily constituent and its related humor both increase or decrease [except in the case of wind where the mode of treatment is the same if wind increases and bone decreases or vice versa.]

This concludes the twenty-ninth chapter, presenting two therapeutic media, from *The Quintessence Tantra, the Secret Oral Tradition of the Eight Branches of the Science of Healing*.

30. Direct Therapeutic Techniques

Then the Sage Rig.pahi.ye.she spoke as follows: O Great Sage, listen.

With regard specifically to treatment of individual imbalances of the three humors: in associated wind disorders sesame oil is supreme [when taken internally, and similarly one should treat the condition] with heavy, oily, smooth, warm-powered dietary factors such as raw cane sugar, grain beer, old butter, mutton stored [for one year], the flesh of marmot, horse, donkey and human, garlic and onion, etc. With respect to behavioral factors one should remain in warm, dim surroundings, hear pleasant speech in attractive company, sleep and wear warm clothing. Regarding medication one should prepare the soup of the three nutritious bones [the tailbone, ankle bone, and shoulder bone of a sheep], and also administer the soup of a complete ram's head which has been preserved for three years, the decoction of the four essences [old meat, matured grain beer, old butter and old cane sugar] and the 'Asafoetida three' decoction. The powders of nutmeg and Asafoetida should also be prescribed and one should prepare the medicinal soups of clarified butter, of mutton, of garlic and of grain beer, the medicinal butters of nutmeg, of garlic, of Aconite, of human bone, of the three (myrobalan fruits) and of the five roots. In short, treatment should be by means of sweet, sour and salty tastes and oily, warm powers. Specifically a warm suppository of old butter is recommended.

As accessory therapy one should massage with one-year-old butter, apply oily fomentations to pain points, and perform moxabustion on the crown of the head, etc., and on the secret wind points. In bile disorders fresh butter is supreme and one should treat with fresh beef and meat of game animals, cool waters, black tea, the curd and buttermilk of cow and goat, porridges of grey and yellow dandelion, of cracked grain, of roasted barley flour and (other) cool (-powered) foods.

The [recommended] behavioral factors entail frequenting breezy places and verdant meadows, sitting under shady trees, remaining undisturbed and relaxing on the banks of rivers or other cool places, and applying cool, fragrant, soothing embrocations.

The three ordinary types of medication are herbal, decoction and selected non-indigenous medicines. According to the strength of a fever one should administer camphor (strongest), [white] sandalwood or animal bile (mildest). In brief one should treat with sweet, bitter and astringent-tasting and cool-powered medication. Specifically sweet-tasting purgatives are recommended. As accessory therapy one should apply sudorifics, avail oneself of a (water) device, let blood from any prominent vein, or apply cold fomentation.

For phlegm disorders (white) honey is supreme. (Moreover) treatment should be by means of mutton, the meat of fish, wild yak, lynx and vulture, as well as by old grain, hot dumplings made from barley flour, matured grain beer, hot boiled water, ginger decoction, etc., and other warm dietary factors in small quantities having light, coarse powers.

With respect to behavioral pattern one should warm oneself by a fire or in the sun, wear warm clothing, exercise oneself mentally and physically in a dry place and abstain from sleeping [during the afternoons].

By way of medication one should administer either salty or hot-tasting concentrated decoctions and compound pomegranate (seeds), *Rhododendron anthopogonoides* with calcinated medicines. In short, one should rely on sour, hot-tasting and light, coarse, and sharp-powered medicines. Specifically sharp, coarse-powered emetics are recommended.

As accessory therapy one should apply fomentations of

[heated] salt, heated lumps of earth or of animal furs. In extremely severe phlegm disorders one should perform moxabustion or (surgical) 'spoon therapy'.

To summarize, wind disorders should be treated by suppository and nutritious factors, bile disorders should be treated by purgation and cool (-powered) factors. In combined wind and bile disorders one should rely on cool, nutritious factors whilst in combined phlegm-bile disorders treatment should be by means of cool, light (-powered) factors. One should treat combined wind and phlegm disorders with warm nutritious factors whilst in triple combined humoral disorders treatment should be by means of cool, nutritious, light factors.

Most essentially all heat disorders should be treated by cool factors whilst all fundamentally cold disorders should be treated as for phlegm. In the case of a combined wind-heat disorder one should treat with oily power, whilst in a cold wind disorder the treatment should be by means of warm-powered factors.

Thus it was said.

This concludes the thirtieth chapter, presenting direct therapeutic techniques, from *The Quintessence Tantra, the Secret Oral Tradition of the Eight Branches of the Science of Healing.*

31. The Healer Physician

Then the Sage Yid.las.skyes spoke as follows: O Teacher, Sage Rig.pahi.ye.she, how should one learn the section on the physician in action? Please expound this, O Healer, King of Physicians.

When he said this the Teacher replied: O Great Sage Yid.las.skyes, the presentation of the section on the active physician, the healer who performs the function of healing, is sixfold: (1) the prerequisites (of a doctor), (2) his nature, (3) his designation, (4) classifications, (5) his function and (6) the results.

THE PREREQUISITES

With respect to the prerequisites, (the doctor) should be (a) intelligent, (b) altruistic, (c) adhering to his words of honor, (d) knowledgeable in practice, (e) diligent, and (f) well-versed in social mores.

Intelligence
Firstly with regard to intelligence, by means of great intellect, stable and cautious attitudes, one should internally actualize all the extensive compilations of therapeutics and thus be without fear of faltering in any practice. By force of such intuitive awareness analytical or extrasensory perception arises which is said to be supreme among the above causes.

Altruism

Altruism entails having an altruistic mind of Enlightenment (which) is threefold: (i) preparation, (ii) performance and (iii) conclusion.

With respect to (i), seeing [that the three realms are in the nature of] suffering, [having the wish to] benefit [sentient beings and having sincere] faith [in the Triple Gem], rather than cling [to notions of] love and hatred [towards others] as being good or bad, by means of even-mindedness [one comes to abide in the four limitless attitudes of] compassion, love, joy, and equanimity.

(ii) (By means of) aspiration [to attain the highest enlightenment for the sake of all sentient beings], the supreme altruistic mind of enlightenment is generated and one should limitlessly engage in this practice.

(iii) (Finally,) in order to actualize this one should thoroughly examine [the application of therapeutics and treat the patients] without prejudice. By having such an attitude the patients will become easier to treat, many will recover and become one's friends.

Adherence to Words of Honor

The adherence to words of honor is said to be threefold: (i) six factors to be kept in mind, (ii) two to be upheld and (iii) three to be understood,

The six factors to be kept in mind are: the preceptor, his teaching, the medical treatises, one's fellow students, the patient, and the latter's pus and blood.

Considering the [preceptor] as the Buddha, [his teaching] as the speech of the rishi ('Upright One'), [the medical treatises] as the Oral Instruction Lineage, [one's fellow students] as friends and relatives, (patients) as one's children, and (their pus and blood) as one's pet dog or pig, are the six words of honor to be preserved.

Two factors to be upheld. Secondly, one should maintain the apprehension of the Medicine Holder of Knowledge as an oath(-bound) protector and his medical instruments as the latter's implements.

Three factors to be understood. Thirdly, medicine is to be understood in a threefold way—as precious gems, as nectar and as offering substances. One should perceive it as a [wish-fulfilling] gem accomplishing one's needs and desires. It should also be perceived as a nectar that dispels diseases and, as the primary offering substance of a Vidhyadhara [Knowledge Holder].

Firstly, these precious medicines should be sought out and retained.

Secondly, it should be well compounded and consecrated [as nectar. The physician] should think of himself as the 'King of Aquamarine Light', consider the medicine container as a begging bowl filled with nectar and [the visualized retinue of] rishis around him as chanting auspiciously.

"O Transcendent Conqueror, Healer King of Physicians, O Medicine Guru Buddha, who dispels the afflictions of the three poisons, whose indigo form [emits] aquamarine light, and whose emanated body is endowed with the major and minor marks; in your right hand you hold a chebulic myrobalan, the antidote to the afflictions of those who are tormented by disorders of wind, bile and phlegm.

"I prostrate to the [one who emits] Aquamarine Light and who holds in his left hand a begging bowl filled with nectar. He has realized the eighteen supreme sciences and has attained the powerful attainment of essence-extraction [which brings] mastery over life itself. I prostrate to the Rishi Vidhyadhara (Sage Knowledge-Holder) [the Supreme Being who balanced collective imbalances of the bodily humors, and who is endowed with clairvoyance and compassion]. To the gods (this medicine) is like nectar, to the serpent spirits like a crowning jewel and to the sages like essence-extraction [-pills]. May this medicine remain ever at the disposal of you (the patients). May it subdue the four hundred and four diseases of wind, bile and phlegm, which threaten life, also subdue the one thousand and eighty types of harmful interferences, the three hundred and sixty intrinsic spirits, etc., and mental obstacles."

> *om namo bhagawate beshajye guru vaidurya prabha rajaya tathagataya arhate sammyaksam buddhaya tadyatha om bheshajye beshajye maha beshajye rajaya samungate svaha*

Having recited [this mantra] seven times one should conceive [the medicine to have been transformed] into nectar. [Having tasted it] one should imagine that by the powerful attainments that have arisen one's afflictions and spirits are dispelled and that by the patient's partaking of it he is relieved (even) of death.

Through upholding (such) words of honor blessings will descend upon one and auspiciousness and merit will ensue.

Knowledge in Practice

Being knowledgeable in practices is threefold: physical, verbal and mental.

[The doctor] should be skilled with his hands at preparing medicines and accessory therapies. He should speak, using sweet words so as to be able to give pleasure to the patient. With regard to mind by means of his bright intellect (the doctor has) clear unmistaken understanding, and one who understands these three is master over all in the aspects of practice.

Diligence

One is diligent with respect to both oneself and others.

Being diligent with respect to oneself (is fourfold): *(a)* one should learn the cause (of becoming a doctor), *(b)* reliance upon [the essential] conditions (e.g., one's teacher), *(c)* diligence with respect to one's fellow students, and *(d)* attainments of consummate familiarization.

(a) With respect to causes one should learn reading and writing to perfection since it is clear [that one's becoming learned] depends on whether one can master these or not.

(b) Relying upon one's preceptor as (the essential) condition is threefold: *(i)* his qualities, *(ii)* the mode of reliance, and *(iii)* the benefit of such reliance.

(i)   One should rely [upon a preceptor], who is extremely learned, endowed with (various) oral instructions, good-natured, of simple means, compassionate and worthy of veneration.

(ii) The mode of reliance: one should entrust oneself (to one's teacher) without harboring doubts about him, perform one's tasks without being two-faced, make all one's actions accord with his will and always maintain the awareness of kindness.

(iii) The advantages (of such) are that one will speedily gain understanding and become learned.

(c) Diligence with respect to one's fellow students: One should ask and put questions [to them about the medical treatises], memorize and contemplate [the meanings thereof] and avoid laziness because this is one's prime obstacle and enemy.

(d) Attainment of consummate familiarization: One should see, hear and absorb [all aspects of medical practice], retain and have intimate knowledge of all such and dispel (all) doubts.

Being diligent with respect to others refers to the patient whom one should treat unstintingly and unwaveringly [until he recovers or is beyond such]. Like someone walking along the top of a (narrow) wall who is threatened with death if he spills [even a drop] from a vessel of melted butter, the doctor should apply assiduous and timely effort in treating by means of medication or accessory therapy.

Social Mores

Being well-versed in social mores is threefold: *(1)* one who is proficient in such, *(2)* one gifted in religious matters, and *(3)* one who is accomplished in both.

With respect to (the first) one should be *(a)* learned and adept [in the codes of conduct that conform to the standards of the world], *(b)* [with one's body, speech and mind do all that is necessary] to be affable and to please (others), and *(c)* subdue them with wrathful means [when necessary]. By these three means [the physician] accomplishes his aims.

(2) If one gifted in religious matters is of subdued disposition, friendly and contented, he will be of benefit to others.

(3) If one is adept in both of the above and maintains compassion for the underprivileged, his essential aims will be fulfilled by the Exalted Ones. One who has these six (prerequisites) will attain (positive) results. Of that there is no doubt.

THE NATURE OF THE DOCTOR

The intimate knowledge of all the characteristics of the [three] humors, the objects of harm [bodily constituents and excretions] and of remedial agents is asserted to be the nature of the physician.

THE DESIGNATION *SMAN.PA*

Because he heals disease and benefits the body (he is called) *sman* (medicine). (He is called *pa* also, since) he is courageous in applying accessory therapy, and also because he is like a father (*pha*) in protecting migrant beings. Because he is held as a lord (*rje*) by kings, the physician (is called *[lha].rje* — Lord of the Gods).

CLASSIFICATIONS

Classifications are threefold: (a) the unsurpassed, (b) superior and (c) ordinary physician.

The Unsurpassed Physician
[The Medicine Buddha] who has overcome the causal three poisons [of attachment, hatred and closed-mindedness] and the resultant [three] humors [of wind, bile and phlegm] is surpassed by none.

The Superior Physician
[The superior physician] is endowed with love and clairvoyant insight into the minds of others, and is upright and true.

The Ordinary Doctor
[The ordinary doctor is of four types:]
(1)   the one of bestowed lineage [who is exhorted to become a physician, e.g., by a religious monarch and who passes on his knowledge to his descendants].
(2)   The one of subsequent learning [who is not a physician of the King but who has gone on to study under such and who has thereby become a doctor].
(3)   One who is familiar with the work [of a physician through having received practical training only.] These

three are friends to sentient beings.

(4) (One who) out of desire [for material gain merely] assumes the guise (of a physician) is a destroyer of life. However, (physicians may be) known as being of superior and inferior types: (the former) should be of noble family, intelligent, abiding by his words of honor, learned in the meanings of the medical texts, having a profound grasp of oral instructions, familiar with medical practice, exert himself principally [in the practice of the Holy] Doctrine and have forsaken desires. [He should also be of] controlled [nature], skilled in practical matters, having a loving attitude towards living beings, diligent, with an outlook [that cherishes] the welfare of others as his own, and unmistaken [in his knowledge of] all the therapies. Such is the superior physician. He is sole protector of suffering beings, the son who upholds the lineage of the Knowledge Holder Sages. I, the emanation of the Healer, King of Physicians, have stated this.

(a) One who lacks such [qualities, who is seen to have] the faults of an inferior doctor and who lacks [a noble] lineage, is like a fox in charge of [a lion's] kingdom. He is neither honored nor respected by anyone.

(b) A 'doctor' who is ignorant of the meanings of the medical texts is like one blind from birth to whom precious substances are shown. [He fails to understand the various] kinds of disease and cannot distinguish the [correct] therapies.

(c) A physician who has neither observed nor acquainted himself [with the practice of a master] is like one who sets out on a new road for the first time. He is assailed by doubts about the symptoms of disease and about the accessory therapies.

(d) The doctor who has no knowledge of diagnostic techniques is like someone wandering in a foreign land without friends or relatives. He cannot recognize a single disease.

(e) The physician who lacks knowledge of pulse and urine diagnosis is like a spy who does not know how to send dispatches. He cannot state even whether a disorder is hot or cold.

(f) A doctor who does not know how to predict [the course that the treatment will take] is like a minister who cannot

express himself properly. He will be affected by disgrace and a poor reputation.

(*g*) The physician who is ignorant of methods of treatment is likened to someone [endeavoring] to strike a target in the dark. The remedy will fail to strike upon the disorder.

(*h*) The doctor who knows nothing of dietary and behavioral factors is like [a ruler] whose country has turned against him. The force of the disease will be increased and the bodily constituents will be suppressed.

(*i*) A physician who is ignorant of pacification compounds is like a farmer who is ignorant about agriculture. Because of insufficient, excess or wrong [compounding] the disorder will be increased.

(*j*) The doctor who is ignorant about purgation is similar to one who pours water on a sandhill. [His treatment] will be unsuited to the disorder and to the bodily constituents.

(*k*) A physician without medical instruments is like a hero bereft of armor or weapons. He will be unable to overcome the enemy of disease and its accompanying factors.

(*l*) Any doctor who is ignorant of venesection and moxabustion is like a burglar who lacks inside information. He will be mistaken with regard to the disorder and the accessory therapy.

Therefore such bad doctors give wrong treatment because of their invariably wrong conceptions. Being demons in the guise of physicians they hold the noose of the Lord of Death and are the lever [which topples the abode] of life. One should not establish any connection (with such doctors) who are the ruin of one's dependents.

THE FUNCTION

The function of a doctor is twofold: ordinary and particular.

Ordinary Function

[The ordinary function of a doctor is threefold according to function of] (i) body, (ii) speech and (iii) mind.

Body. Physically he amasses the [necessary] medicinal ingredients and instruments and strives for the patient's welfare.

Speech. The function of his speech is to predict [the course of the patient's treatment] and through his realizing [the nature of the disorder] he can pronounce such in the manner of blowing a conch in the market place. [The physician] should either guarantee the patient's survival or [discreetly] announce the time of his passing. If he cannot determine [the nature of] the disorder he should make ambiguous pronouncements like the tongue of a snake. Thus being astride either [possibility the physician] should then have recourse to whichever is the more positive pronouncement.

Otherwise [if both the doctor and patient] are agreed about the apparent [nature of the disorder then the former should clearly express this to the latter].   Once the physician is convinced [of the nature of the disorder] he should still [outwardly] agree with the patient's opinion [whilst prescribing according to what he has ascertained the disorder to be]. When the avenues of [different] possibilities are open [then the doctor can] retire [safely] to the fortress [of the stable pronouncements that he has made].

(a) In the first case, if the doctor realizes the condition to be as the patient suspects then, agreeing with the latter, he should express clearly that the disorder is indeed the same.

(b) In the second case the patient may suspect (his problem to be) poisoning and the physician diagnoses otherwise. Since it is possible [that the patient may] denounce [the doctor as being unskilled], because the latter has not concurred on the basis of what the patient believes, [the doctor should manifest] agreement and, having [thoroughly] examined the syndrome, he should treat the disorder as it actually is.

(c) Thirdly, whether the patient will survive, whether death threatens, whether the danger is great or small, are (all) influenced by the [four] conditions of the 'good fortune', the karma, power and merit (of both the doctor and patient). Since he may die or may survive the physician cannot make predictions with absolute clarity. Even though the danger may be great the physician may still state that a cure [is feasible] and (even) if there is little danger one should stress the necessity of taking (great) care [of the patient's condition]. Moreover one should conform with the customs [and accepted standards] of the world.

Mind. With respect to mental function the doctor should examine unerringly, thoroughly and with much deliberation. Particular function is threefold: *(a)* view, *(b)* familiarization and *(c)* conduct.

Regarding *view*, (the physician) should have realized (the View) of the Middle Way with respect to all phenomena and by means of this supreme view, the perfect view of the Middle Way he should have abandoned the extremes of inferiority, of excess and of error.

With regard to *familiarization* one should abide by the Four Immeasureables. It is imperative not to lose oneself down any of the four 'wrong turnings' of:

(i)   pampering ungrateful patients and therefore affording less attention to other patients,

(ii)   overdoing compassion for those who have hatred for the Holy Doctrine or sentient beings,

(iii) feeling joy when the patients of other doctors pass away,

(iv)   being indifferent to whether patients live or die.

Of the two types of *conduct*, i.e., that which is to be adopted and that which is to be abandoned, one should abandon non-virtues. (Specifically) one should refrain from deluded conduct, talking nonsense, 'showing off', harmful and negative actions.

[With regard to conduct to be adopted,] one should practice generosity, ethics, patience and energy, (as well as concentration and wisdom).

THE RESULTS
The results of being a physician are temporal and ultimate.

Temporal Results
Temporally in this life one will be endowed with happiness, influence, prosperity, joy and bliss. One achieves these through Medicine and one should display one's qualities to others. Harmful people should be treated affectionately like relatives. They should be examined, checked thoroughly and treated in accordance with their behavioral pattern. By force of practicing in this way one will win merit and renown, and the food and possessions one wishes will appear.

At these times one should be modest and apply (what one has learned). When one is in demand one should accept food, money or measures (of grain, etc.), for if this is deferred (then later when the patient has) forgotten the kindness rendered to him (by the doctor) he will offer nothing to repay him.

Ultimate Results

With respect to ultimate results, a physician who has abandoned deceit and desire and who engages in healing will proceed to the unsurpassed state of Buddhahood.

This has been stated by the Healer, King of Physicians. Having thus spoken, (the sage) Rig.pahi.ye.she dissolved back into the crown protrusion of the King of Medicine.

This concludes the thirty-first chapter, on the healer physician, from *The Quintessence Tantra, the Secret Oral Tradition of the Eight Branches of the Science of Healing.*

The Explanatory Tantra of *The Quintessence Tantra, the Secret Oral Tradition of the Eight Branches of the Science of Healing* is here concluded.

Notes

THE ROOT TANTRA

Chapter 1

1. The deva disciples heard 'The Healing Therapy Vase,'
    The rishis heard 'Charaka Astanga,'
    The non-Buddhists heard the 'Tantra of Black Mahadeva,'
    The Buddhists heard 'The Circle of the Lords of the Three Families.'

2. This refers specifically to the sage Yid.las.skyes.

Chapter 2

1. Inflamed swellings of microbes, in the blood from birth, that react with wind, bile and phlegm, including swelling of arms, legs and throat.

2. Twenty types especially caused by phlegm and including diabetes, e.g., the excess build up of sweet substances in the body which gives rise to parasites. The latter should be treated with Embelia.

3. Red, itchy, inflamed sores of developed blood, bile and fluid.

4. In which blood or waste fluids, e.g., lymph, create tumors in the ducts of the organs; suppuration also occurs.

5.   In which blood and lymph descend and cause swelling in the legs.

6.   Nagas are serpent-spirits.

7.   These are especially for hot disorders, e.g., desiccated decoction stored in a sheep's stomach.

8.   For example, to pound gold, silver, copper and iron as thin as bees' wings and put in a sealed vessel in a cow-dung fire.

Chapter 5

1.   The best type is of a hero who died in battle, but the flesh of any violent person would suffice.

THE EXPLANATORY TANTRA

Chapter 3

1.   A transparent blue and white gem.

Chapter 4

1.   All measurements quoted here are according to the individual person's dimensions and not as measured by the doctor.

Chapter 6

1.   We have to revise this estimate downwards nowadays.

Chapter 7

1.   *Ichug.ma* is a plant with large sour-tasting leaves and stalk like those of a turnip.

Chapter 16

1.   A dzo is a yak crossed with a cow.

2.   Sanskrit: *chilli.*

3.   Sanskrit: *krakalasah.*

4. Sections (c) and (d) are here counted as one.

5. *Chenopodium album.*

6. Mon variety of *Chenopodium.*

Chapter 20

1. Sanskrit: *himavat.*

2. Sanskrit: *vinvya.*

3. A type of bird.

4. Turkestan.

5. Serpent spirits.

6. A jagged rock which fragments into spearhead-shaped pieces.

7, 8. Great Tibetan scholar-physicians of the past.

9. Lit. 'skygoers,' a type of altruistic female celestial.

10. Nyctalopia: a type of blindness.

11. The great patriarch of Tibetan medicine, gYu.thog Yon.ten mGon.po.

12. Section 6, "Exposition of the Powers of Plants," does not appear as a separate section in the original text; nor is there agreement among scholars and commentators through the ages about which substances should be included in this section.

13. *chhig.thub.dkar.po*: a generic name referring to plants having a unique power to heal disease without being compounded with other substances.

14. *chu.ser.lhog.pa*, tuberculous lymph nodes which discharge into the skin.

15. There are twenty-five different types of *dar.ya.kan.*

16. *sur.ya*: metastatic cancer.

17. Tib. *hbyung.po*, pronounced 'jung-po'.

Chapter 21

1.   *tsi.stag* is equivalent to *chhu.ma.rtsi.*

Chapter 26

1.   This paragraph describes the qualities of an ideal patient who would be easiest to treat.

Chapter 28

1.   "The four waters": a figurative usage referring to the cool power that all four remedial factors have in common.

General Index

A

Commiphora mukul   146
Common Fumitory   164, 184
Conch shell   132
Conesi   126
Copper   131
Coptis teetoides   166
Coral   133
Corallodiscus   168
Corallodiscus kingianus   166,
   185
Coriander   144, 185, 215
Coriandrum sativum   144
Corn Smut   172
Corydalis edulis   126, 156, 184
Corydalis meifolia   171
Costus root   150, 185
Costus speciosus   150
Cow urine   181
Cowhage   149
Cowrie shell   178
Crab   182, 186
Crag halite   147
Crane   25, 112
Cremanthodium   116
Crocodile   181
Crocus sativus   141
Croton tiglium   154, 175
Crystal Orb (text)   13
Crystal Rosary (text)   13, 15, 17
Cuculus canorus   112
Cuculus melanoleucus   179
Cuminum cymimum   142
Curcuma longa   151
Curcurbita pepo   155
Cuscuta europaea   165
Cuscuta sinensis   160
Cynanchum sibiricum   143
Cyrtiospirifer sinensis   134

D

Dalbergia lanceolaria   169
Dandelion   37, 115, 221
Daphne odora   163
Daphne tangutica   185

Date   150
Datura   185
Datura alba   163
Datura stramonium   163
Daucus carota   165
Debregeasia edulus   152
Deer blood   180
Deer fat   180
Delphinium brunonianum
   158
Delphinium cashmirianum
   158
Delphinium grandiflorum   174,
   186
Delphinium viscosum   174
Dendrobium curcuminatum
   151
Dianthus superbus   158
Dill   162
Dilmar Geshe Tenzin Phuntsok
   13
Diptheria   29, 94, 97
Dockleaf   171
Dog stool   182
Dog testicle   179
Dog tongue   179
Donkey   181
Donkey blood   180
Donkey tongue   179
Dontostemon pectinatus   172
Draba alata   172
Draba nemorosa   158
Dracocephalum tangutium   156
Dragon bone   178
Drynaria propinqua   168
Dryopteris fragrans   166
Duck, Red Wild   112, 180
Dung beetle   182
Dyer's Madder   169

E

Eaglewood   38, 107, 140, 185
Echinops   174
Eczema   93

Index of Tibetan Names